# Decoding The Body's Messages

*Unlock Your Wisdom To Heal*

Rachel Claire Farnsworth

To my gorgeous son & daughter George and Emily. My life is so enriched because of you both. I love you beyond words.

Special thanks to Francis Carl Adlaon for designing the cover, Janine Kathleen Shapiro & Laura Shofroth for your support, collaboration and contributions.

Thank you, Jemma Collins, for proofreading and writing the foreword in the book. I appreciate you so very much.

*Healing at your personal root cause is the master padlock and the real master key is self love.*

*Rachel C Farnsworth*

## About the Author

Rachel Claire Farnsworth, a 5 times award-winning Transformational & Wellness Therapist and Trauma Releasing Expert, has been instrumental in helping clients worldwide achieve their health and wellness goals. Her journey began when she successfully used hypnotherapy to help her daughter overcome an autoimmune disease, leading her to develop her own Decode Root Cause Method.

Rachel is an internationally best-selling author, having co-authored three books. Her recent accolades include The Global Health Pharma award for her contributions to mental health and the title of Trauma Releasing Specialist for Central England, further solidifying her expertise and dedication to her field.

Her clients have given her the title 'Spiritual Midwife' because releasing trauma allows you to come back to your true soul essence. It is the meaning of true self love.

# *Foreword*

I first met Rachel in 2019 when, by the smallest of chances, we came across each other's paths when I was working in a job that I only had for 3 months. Upon meeting her, it was clear how kind and empathetic she was. I knew nothing about the work she was embarking upon at the time, but I knew somewhere in the back of my subconscious mind that our lives would continue down a path where we would work together again in the future.

She showed empathy to me, and her kind nature immediately made me feel at ease and I opened up to her about some traumatic events from my past that only very few people knew, and certainly not things I'd usually share with someone I had only just met. However, something deep down told me how trustworthy she was, and I immediately felt at ease in her presence, comfortable sharing some of my darkest times.

With a career and personal history based in the medical and scientific field, I would have considered myself a sceptic if you had asked me about Rachel's field of work at the beginning of 2019. Her wonderful and kind personality glows through everything she does and says, and we remained friends ever since. She offered to work with me many times between our meeting in 2019 to the point where it finally happened in 2024. On previous occasions, I just never felt ready to embark on that journey but both of us agreed that we both knew that one day the stars would align, and we would be able to work together. Everyone with past trauma knows that going over past events can be upsetting and also not knowing how it worked made me shy away from reaching out for help.

When we finally set the date to work together for my first session, I was so nervous. I didn't know what to expect. I didn't want to have any expectations at all for fear of feeling like I've failed or let Rachel down. I have Borderline Personality Disorder and OCD, so these thoughts are something I battled with daily. I live in a black and white world, with no grey areas, no room to accept other viewpoints, very low self-esteem, very traumatic past abuse during my childhood, adolescent years and also into adulthood at the hands of previous partners. I had no idea what Rachel's technique even involved and when I told a friend about 'hypnotherapy', jokes were made about her making me cluck like a chicken in the stereotypical vision of hypnotherapy that we all have.

I was provided with a personal recording to listen to for a week prior to the first session which prepared me and enabled me to learn how to relax, something I had never been able to do. I never ever fully relaxed. I had tension all over my body. I had deep depression, severe anxiety, very severe attachment and abandonment issues, trust issues, trauma, a painful neck and shoulder, fear of being out of control and a general feeling of unease at just being alive and existing on a daily basis.

Once I had learned to relax, we had our first session. My subconscious mind took me to places I did not expect it to take me to. I expected it to take me to really obvious traumatic events that I can recount well but instead I was given scenes in my subconscious mind I had forgotten about. Trauma is a funny thing, and our brains are rewired to forget these events but yet we still live in fear, in fight or flight mode. Rachel's technique brought forward some past events and Rachel talked me through how to let these events go, how to heal my inner child and help the child at the time of these events and build up my self-confidence and resilience and realise that nothing was my fault.

I was able to let go of some really upsetting history and terrible times of my life. Afterwards, I felt relaxed and tired for the rest of the day but proud of myself for sticking with it. I was then given another personal recording from Rachel to listen to after the session to reaffirm what we had covered.

Rachel reached back out to me to check in to see if I needed another session, but I actually felt like I didn't need one. I felt light. I felt freer. I have not had a single panic attack since the day of our session. Things that would previously trigger me have melted into insignificance. A calmness had washed over me which was the most bizarre feeling as I had not had this feeling since the day I was born probably! I'd find myself thinking, 'hmm usually I'd be panicking about this situation' but yet, there I was, stoic in my approach and calm and with this unfamiliar feeling of clarity and calmness. I've since enjoyed time on my own, away from my husband, which previously would have been a huge trigger for my abandonment issues. I approach challenges with my parenting with a different, more patient attitude. My neck and shoulder issue has not troubled me since.

I honestly feel like I've released the burden and the tension inside my body. I am no longer living in turmoil. I no longer see myself as someone unworthy of love. I no longer overthink every single scenario. I no longer hate myself. I no longer think I am a burden to people. I no longer have suicidal thoughts.

I am an amazing, clever, funny, kind, loving person, deserving of love and affection. If it wasn't for that chance meeting with Rachel and her empathy and skill at recognising someone in turmoil, I don't know where I would be. As I stated previously, I am a huge sceptic with a scientific and medical-based job and used to consider this type of intervention as 'woo woo'. I can honestly say it has been life changing for me.

I know other traumatic events may occur in my life and previous events may resurface, but I know that Rachel will always be there for further sessions if I need them, and for now, I am just happy that I can adopt a different approach to my life. My main goal was to just be able to live in the moment, and allow myself to be happy and I think I'm finally on the road to the life I deserve.

Thank you for everything Rachel. You deserve all the success and recognition you have achieved thus far and will continue to receive in the future. Your work is of great importance, and I hope you realise just how vital people like you are in this hardened, tough world. Thank you for asking me to work with you on this new book. You're an absolute inspiration.

With much love,

Jemma

# Contents

# *Introduction*

'Decoding The Body's Messages' is a heartfelt invitation to begin to untangle the pattern of pain and symptoms. My desire for you is to begin to understand what your body tells you, to be able to listen to its messages and to unlock the wisdom to heal you.

We all face challenges, and we as a family, had been going through the ordeal of trying the best we could to manage my daughter's symptoms of her autoimmune disease. Emily, my daughter, had been diagnosed with Juvenile Idiopathic Arthritis (JIA) in 2005 when she was just eighteen months old. We noticed that she was walking oddly by throwing her left leg out, and her joints were swollen and puffy. She was diagnosed a few months later and we had been following doctors' advice since her diagnosis. Emily was having regular blood tests and scans and was taking a cocktail of medication, including steroid injections and methotrexate.

While the medication kept the symptoms at bay, it also gave her plenty of additional symptoms. Her side effects included poor memory, being withdrawn and was very sick every weekend when she self-injected the drugs she had been prescribed. She fell ill with every cough and cold going around as the drugs compromised her immune system. She took the medication at weekends, which meant she was violently sick every Saturday; she felt completely washed out on Sundays and back to school on Mondays. It was no family life for any of us. She had countless hospital trips, steroid injections, blood tests, and scans too. We were regularly at the hospital and, at the time, believed this was the best way to help my daughter.

Isn't it curious how the universe works, though? Every time we attended the hospital for routine appointments and steroid injections, it seemed that 'Fix You' by Coldplay was on the radio. I would sing the line 'I will fix you' with tears cascading down my face and a silent prayer to the universe that if there is a solution, please can it present itself to me, as I have no idea where to begin to look.

In the background of all that was happening with Emily, in June 2018, I became a certified practitioner in advanced hypnotherapy just because the subject interested me. Hypnotherapy is a natural state of relaxation that allows us to be more in our subconscious mind, which is 95% of everything we do, think, feel, and believe about ourselves. It is also our emotional mind and where our memories are stored.

In July 2018, Emily was now 14 and had been in drug-induced remission for 2 whole years. The doctors were hopeful that she may have outgrown the disease. We were ecstatic at this prospect. She came off the drugs as they advised, and just eight weeks later she experienced a flare-up of the disease once more. We were heartbroken. The doctors advised her to go back on the drugs and not to be surprised if what she required was even stronger medication than before. We were distraught to say the very least.

Emily and I decided to have a hypnotherapy session together in October of 2018, when her flare-up started, to see if we could use my new skills in a desperate attempt to help her at least reduce some of the pain and symptoms she experienced daily.

It wasn't my best session because it was my first. I also hadn't understood the link between our emotional and physical symptoms back then either. Nevertheless, to our surprise and delight, we were able to find her personal unique root cause. Our session together revealed that she subconsciously believed that she needed the pain to be like her cousins, her brother, and myself, as we all had pain and symptoms of our own at the time she was diagnosed. Once she could understand it consciously, she was able to release it in that single session. She has had no pain, no symptoms and no medication ever since.

That session empowered my daughter, without a doubt. However, it also sparked a passion in me to help others because we had been stuck in that never-ending cycle of pain, symptoms, and suffering for fourteen years, and now I had a powerful tool to help others free themselves.

It ignited something in me to unravel the mysteries of our body and its messages. Our bodies whisper and sometimes shout secrets to us, waiting for us to listen and decode them patiently. The body is the link between the subconscious and conscious minds. Pain and symptoms are simply messages requesting we go within and release the hidden and suppressed emotions lying behind them.

As you read through the pages of this book, I hope you will begin to understand what is happening in your body. I invite you to read this book with an open and inquisitive mind. Be willing to entertain the possibility that chronic pain and your symptoms have deeper messages waiting to be understood.

Your body isn't broken, it is brilliantly trying to communicate with you. Together through these pages, I want to help you explore what is going on for you. While not every ailment or condition can be covered, I hope you will see what is going on within your body, see the truth about health and genetics, shine a light on the interconnectedness of emotions, beliefs, thoughts, and your physical health, as the mind, body, spirit is inseparably linked.

Although your healing journey is uniquely yours, you do not need to walk it alone. 'Decoding The Body's Messages' is more than just a guide; it is a path to wellness as there are chapters dedicated to helping you help yourself to the potential for healing that resides within you. Trust that your body knows how to heal given the right circumstances.

We have an infinite intelligence, a consciousness, which

runs through us. If you accidentally cut yourself, your body knows how to heal that cut; you don't need to give it any conscious thought. In the same way, we don't really need to think about breathing, or our heart pumping blood around our bodies. Cell repair and renewal happen continually yet we are blissfully unaware of the process. Women don't need to think about how to grow a baby, their bodies automatically know how to do it. In the same way, your body knows how to heal given the right circumstances.

Your body isn't broken; it simply conveys a message. Once the message is understood, the physical symptoms can and do disappear.

I will help you release and dispel any preconceived ideas that you may have, such as 'our health is genetic,' that 'random pain and symptoms occur with no apparent cause' and that our 'bodies malfunction for no reason and there's little or nothing we can do about it.'

Right now, you, or someone you know, are probably struggling with a diagnosis of anxiety, depression, PTSD, an autoimmune disease, or other chronic illness or condition. These symptoms are likely to affect your relationships, you may feel like your life has been put on hold because you can no longer do the things you'd love to, or previously enjoyed. The symptoms will likely affect your overall happiness, career, relationships, and bank balance because your potential earnings have been diminished. Let's begin to change that now.

Within these pages, you will gain a deeper understanding of what your body tells you. Then, I will help you release your current negative thoughts and beliefs and replace them with healthier ones. You can download and listen to several self-help tools, and I am confident you will enjoy them. The book contains lots of free resources and additional ones you can purchase if you wish to take your healing to a deeper level.

So, let's start the journey together. As you read this book with a curious, open mind, I intend that you will see and understand how powerful you truly are and find the solutions you seek.

Together, we will walk toward a life defined not by pain and anxiety but by understanding, optimal wellness, and joy.

Welcome to the beginning of your life transformation.

Much Love

*Rachel*

# *Setting Our Intentions*

A few years ago, I may have laughed at the title of this section or rolled my eyes internally because I didn't realise that our thoughts create our reality.

I have come to realise that the intentions behind our actions count and make a huge difference to the outcomes we are seeking, simply because our energy is our real currency. Energy flows where our attention goes, so let's consciously start by setting what you seek within this book so that it has the power to make a huge difference and shift in your life.

I, therefore, create this space and time for us both to set our intentions for the book.

You will notice I have left a few lines for you to write your intentions so that you can revisit them and even alter them again if you wish to.

I intend to help dispel any preconceived ideas about illness and disease.

I will show you that we don't have random pain and symptoms, there is an emotional root cause – I have worked on thousands of sessions with clients and every single one has had an emotional root.

We don't have to live with pain and symptoms; our bodies have an inborn, natural ability to heal.

Later in the book, after we explore pain and symptoms, there are tools and techniques, including guided meditations, to help you achieve optimal health and true wellness.

I break the steps down into simple parts so that you can understand what the missing ingredient is and help yourself. The answers will probably astound you. I am keeping it simple because it is simple. You just haven't been shown until now.

Now it is your turn to take a few moments to reflect on what you hope to gain from this book and what you hope to achieve. Allow yourself to think big because you are more powerful than you have been led to believe.

_____

_____

_____

_____

_____

_____

_____

_____

_____

_____

_____

_____

_____

_____

_____

_____

_____

_____

_____

_____

_____

_____

_____

_____

_____

_____

_____

_____

_____

_____

I wish you every amazing thing you wish for yourself and so much more.

# *Awakening To Our True Essence*

B efore I go deeper into the topic of healing, I believe it is important for us to comprehend who or what we are, so you have some concept of how powerful you truly are. You are so much more than just a body with some thoughts running through your head. You are a multi-dimensional consciousness. You are an energetic being having a human experience. It is impossible to kill energy, it simply transforms. Think of ice becoming water, steam, and vapour.

Your soul came into your body to experience the human experience and learn certain lessons along the way. Think of it like an individually set exam paper; you have unique tasks and challenges along the way, which is why there's no point comparing yourself to others. You have your distinct fingerprints expressing life in your own unique way.

Our consciousness doesn't die, only our body does. When I was small, I used to have fleeting flashbacks like I was being pulled upwards, almost like being pulled up along a rope, and a conversation took place that felt as though it was in a higher place. Over time these images have become slightly clearer. I believe that I was accessing a memory as I was incarnating into this lifetime. I think this was when I was in the womb, and I was negotiating the terms of being here. I have a 'knowing' that it was agreed that I was going to incarnate with another soul, so we were together from the beginning of this lifetime, but this changed as I was in the womb and already committed. When I was about to be born, I was trying to come feet first and was born by caesarean. Every birthday, Mum retold the story that I didn't know how to be born as I was feet first. My take on this was that if I didn't know how to be born, I shouldn't be on the planet. That gave me lots of anxiety and a feeling of being an imposter. I have read books that teach that being feet first is a reluctance to come into the world. That feels true for me.

My son, when he was very young and first began to learn to talk, often cried for his 'other mother, not you, mummy,' he would sob. I would have gladly taken him to her as he was so distraught. These memories and my hypnotherapy sessions, as a client, and as a therapist, have made me believe beyond doubt that we are eternal beings having a human experience. I have experienced past and in-between lives myself during these sessions.

Even when you were in the womb, you were picking up other people's emotions, particularly your mother's, as you were being bathed in her emotions, just as the rest of her body was absorbing everything she thought and felt. When you realise that the eggs in a female's body are created as the embryo is being developed, you can see that part of you was actually being formed in your grandmother's body when your mother was developing. From this alone, you can begin to see how trauma is passed down through the generations.

Your mind is like a sponge absorbing the world around you. When you were small, you had very little life experience and were unable to question what you saw and believed. You just absorbed it all. This is when thoughts and beliefs about yourself and the outside world are formed, and these thoughts and beliefs stay with you until you become aware of them and decide to change them; some are positive experiences, and others are not.

As soon as you are born, you adopt many beliefs and opinions about how the world works through your environment, music, TV, school, family, caregivers, and friends. We are led to believe that we are simply humans who need to go to school, college, work, maybe get married, and have children.

This is how we assume life is, and we share collective beliefs on how the world works. We are not taught in school that we are energetic beings, or how to use our energy. Instead, we are told to use our logical mind through English and Maths or anything analytical to keep us in our heads so that we are disassociated from our bodies and our true selves and just believe everything we see.

You elected to come down into your human body to experience it physically through your senses. You are here to experience contrasts, different emotions and sensations to help your soul grow and evolve. The problem is that you become bogged down by other people's opinions of you, and seduced and taken in by the material and physical world. You forget who you really are, and all too soon, the belief that 'I am not enough' takes hold of you and becomes one of your core beliefs that stays with you as a 'truth' until you question it and release it.

The truth is you don't just have a soul, you *are* a soul. For many of us though, the soul feels hidden, and you may not even realise or acknowledge that you have a higher power or are even aware you are a vital part of the web of creation.

We are energetic beings, and as you cannot kill energy; it just shifts and changes form, this must mean that we are eternal beings having a human experience. Pretty much every system in our world is hiding the truth of who we really are.

What happens is that your soul seems to shout louder with its messages the further you deviate away from your true soul self.

Anxiety, depression, or other long-term health issues and diseases are your body's way of telling you that you are out of alignment or separated from who you truly are. You feel out of alignment because of the experiences that made you feel bad about yourself.

Your soul may feel hidden because of the limiting and restricting beliefs that you hold to be true about yourself. These beliefs were formed through traumas you experienced. Trauma is any situation or event that makes you feel bad about yourself.

# *Exploring the Subconscious Mind*

T he subconscious mind is one of the most fascinating and least understood areas of the human psyche. Sigmund Freud was the first person to introduce us to the idea of the unconscious mind, laying the foundations for others to conduct their own discoveries and research. I am not going to discuss the historical discoveries here, instead, we are going to investigate together how the subconscious impacts your life and the lives of others you care about.

The subconscious mind is 95% of your thoughts, actions and reactions that are unconscious but are apparent through your reality. The subconscious shapes your world so much without your conscious awareness. The subconscious mind is a treasure trove, waiting to be unlocked, holding the keys to your deepest fears, greatest aspirations, and untapped potentials. It's where creative inspiration whispers, and solutions to your problems suddenly emerge, crystal clear, into the light. The beauty of this hidden realm is that it's intimately connected with every one of us, guiding you and shaping your actions.

Take a look at your life right now, for it is a reflection, a mirror of what your subconscious believes. This isn't just philosophy, it's a profound truth that I am passionate about exploring with you. The subconscious mind is the gateway to your higher self, where you can access all the answers you seek.

Only 5% of your mind is conscious thoughts. If your conscious mind is such a tiny part of your mental state, I think you can start to see how powerful your subconscious mind is. It's the silent puppeteer, pulling strings and shaping your life in ways you seldom recognise because it is all done without conscious thinking.

Every area of your life, from your financial status, your health, and your relationships with yourself and others, is shaped not by your conscious decisions but by a force much deeper and more powerful. That force is your subconscious.

Have you ever noticed the pattern in how you approach different aspects of your life? It appears that 'how you do one thing is how you do everything.' This isn't just a coincidence. It's a reflection of your subconscious programming in action. This hidden architect has been designing the blueprint of your life, often without your conscious permission.

Much of this programming was etched into your mind when you were a small child, young, impressionable, and not fully capable of independent thought or decision-making. Therefore, an astonishing 95% of your life is not steered by your conscious self but is directed backstage by your subconscious, creating habits and beliefs like puppet strings that control the outcomes of your days and your life.

When you were a child, you were dependent on others to take care of you, so it was paramount for you to fit into your surroundings for your survival. That is why the fear of rejection is so strong. If you really got rejected it could seriously have impacted your chance of survival. There is a deep-seated fear of rejection because you would be less likely to be able to survive on your own. As you mature and become an adult, there is a need to look at that subconscious programming because those old ways no longer benefit you. As a child, you needed to fit in. As an adult, you need to stand out, so there is a disconnect between your thoughts and beliefs. That is partly why growing up can feel so difficult and often gives you that push-pull feeling in your mind. It is that tug of war between your conscious thinking and your subconscious programming.

Your subconscious mind is not logical, it is emotional. That is why, in a situation where emotion versus logic, emotions will almost always win because it is the language of the subconscious mind. The subconscious is also where memories are stored, and that is why you get triggered. Imagine a filing cabinet in your mind where past situations are filed away by emotion rather than chronological dates. It is also why you may have anxiety and panic attacks because past events are triggering your responses in the now and current moments.

Your subconscious mind does not understand the past, present and future, it only understands the right here, right now moment because time does not exist the same way you experience it. Therefore, the subconscious doesn't understand that what happened in the past is unlikely to happen again. It hasn't grasped that the bullies in school won't appear around the corner, or that you left school years ago. It doesn't understand that you have moved on so much since you were younger. It is still building and creating your now moment from past experiences and events. It is also why your mind will give you every excuse it can to stop you from doing something new because it wants to keep you in the familiar patterns so it can keep you 'safe' in the remits it is familiar with.

There are certain characteristics our subconscious minds have. It will resist you if your conscious mind is trying too hard. For example, if you are trying to think of a person's name and you are concentrating hard trying to remember, you will probably notice that the more you try, the more it alludes you. However, if you say instead, that thought or name will come back to me, you will notice that you remember so much quicker.

Every thought you think creates a physical and emotional response. Your thoughts create chemicals which, in turn, have a huge influence on your physical body. The chemicals in your brain allow your body to feel what you are thinking. If you think a happy thought, your brain is likely to produce more thoughts that make you feel more inspired and joyful, and then the chemical dopamine is released which will give you feelings of pleasure and satisfaction in your body and is likely to inspire you to be more motivated which also helps increase your memory and concentration and improve your sleep patterns.

Equally hateful, angry, or other more negative thoughts will create a physical response. You may become aware of your body feeling tense, maybe that tight, familiar anxious knot in your stomach. Thinking creates feeling. Feeling creates thinking, and it is a perpetual cycle. These feelings and thoughts create a state in the body that becomes your default setting for how you think and behave.

Your mind loves the familiar and has been conditioned to a certain way of thinking all your life. It will try to keep you where you are because it cannot predict your future; it only knows what it already knows. It will do all it can and give you lots of excuses for why you need to stay in your comfort zone. If you desire change, feel the fear and do it anyway.

No matter what you tell yourself, your subconscious mind will believe it, regardless of whether it is a positive or negative thought. I am fat, ugly stupid, or I am pretty, smart, and loveable. It doesn't matter, your mind will take it in as a truth. Start today and say positive things about yourself and keep doing it because your mind learns by repetition. Your mind cannot hold conflicting beliefs either, they simply cancel each other out.

Your life is a masterful tapestry, woven with threads of beliefs that subconsciously guide you. But are you standing in your creation with a sense of fulfilment, or do you find yourself yearning for more? Your subconscious beliefs are the silent architects of your reality. These foundational, core beliefs about yourself create your external world and how you perceive your place within it. These beliefs often stem from early childhood experiences and societal frameworks and have been etched deeply into the fabric of your being.

But here's the catch: Many of us walk through life not knowing that we're holding on to these beliefs, much less questioning their validity or how they shape our existence. It's as if we're running an outdated operating system, complete with bugs and glitches that no longer serve us.

Isn't it strange to think that we are so quick and willing to change our laptops, or our mobile phones and update them with the latest technology, yet hardly ever pay the attention we perhaps should to our own internal software, in our own subconscious mind. When was the last time you re-wired your own internal software?

If you recognise the disconnect between your desires and your reality, it's a sign that it's time to decode the programming that runs beneath the surface, time to question if these beliefs align with the person you aspire to be or are holding you back.

You can begin by asking yourself some fundamental questions:

- What stories have I been subscribing to without questioning?
- Where did these beliefs originate, and who gave them to me?
- Where did I acquire them from?
- Do these beliefs limit or empower me?

Analysing your subconscious beliefs isn't just an academic exercise, it's an act of reclaiming the power over your own life's script.

Here's the empowering part: Once you recognise the immense influence of your subconscious, you can begin to take the reins back. You can reprogram your mind and reshape your life towards the success and fulfilment you yearn for and deserve.

To change your life, you have to change your thoughts and beliefs both in your conscious and subconscious minds. Just doing it consciously is like driving a car with the handbrake on as your subconscious will keep pulling you back into the old familiar patterns. Your subconscious mind is your personal thermostat ensuring you reach your default points in all areas of your life.

Being aware of what is going on is key to change.

Awareness is the first step, otherwise, it remains in your blind spot. You have to make these things conscious before you can make the necessary changes.

It's part of our human experience to grow and evolve, to experience contrasts that help us dismantle limiting beliefs and construct empowering ones. You're not just a witness to your transformation, you're the conductor.

Your future is brimming with possibilities. The past does not dictate the horizon of your opportunities. When you make a conscious effort to analyse and alter your inner programming, you don't just change a belief; you unlock a new level of self-awareness. When your inner world changes, your outer world does as well, bringing about lots of new experiences. Here's to your rebirth, to a future forged by creating helpful life-changing beliefs. You are becoming the conscious programmer of your own life, and the next chapter promises to be nothing short of remarkable.

# Our Core Beliefs & Deep Seated Needs

In the previous chapter, we discussed the workings of the subconscious mind and its undeniable influence over us. Your beliefs either serve you as stepping stones or stumbling blocks. The truth is that if you believe that you can or cannot accomplish a task, you're right in both cases.

Let's take a deeper look into what helps shape and form your beliefs about yourself and the world around you. Your beliefs came from your met and unmet needs as you were growing up.

From your earliest moments, you were trying to make sense of the world around you, and your emotions played a big part in this as they are your navigational system, your compass. In the same way your sense of touch allows you to understand if something is soft, hard, hot, cold, rough, or smooth.

Your perception of your self-worth is a core foundation that underpins your image of who you believe you are. Most of us walk through life carrying the weight of 'not being enough', a sentiment deeply wounding and engraved by past experiences particularly when you were small and making sense of the world around you.

Your core beliefs revolve around the three basic needs that each of us requires to thrive:

**Boundaries:**

The ability to assert 'yes' or 'no' is a crucial aspect of autonomy. Healthy boundaries are about being able to make your decisions about what to do in a situation without being influenced by someone else or being told what to do. It allows you to convey your preferences both to yourself and to other people. Saying 'yes' when you mean 'no,' or the other way around, can make you feel you have compromised yourself because you haven't paid enough care for your own needs and wants and have tried to meet someone else's needs first instead of your own.

**Safety:**

From your earliest moments, your sense of safety is regulated through your interactions with those entrusted to care for you. This underpins your ability to regulate your emotions and navigate the world confidently or with anxious thoughts and a lack of self-belief.

**Love:**

The essence of love is really about feeling cherished just for being who you are and not for what you do. If you aren't loved unconditionally as a child, it can lead to patterns of being the rescuer, the high achiever, the helper, the sick child, and/or the naughtier/difficult child. Which role(s) did you learn to play and why did you learn to take on that role? It is often because that was the only way you received attention or felt loved.

In the hustle of achieving, helping, and adapting, you probably received mixed signals, leading to deep-seated patterns that compromised your self-worth.

# *Understanding Trauma*

T he term trauma often conjures up images of abuse, neglect and devastating experiences that unequivocally alter lives. It spans from physical harm and suffering to emotional deprivation and household instability, all of which implant seeds of enduring emotional and often physical pain. These events cause internal conflicts and wounds within yourself which we will discuss.

Beyond the more obvious traumas, let's recognise the covert trauma which is more subtle. These are experiences of not being seen, not being heard, not feeling cherished or loved. We have all had these instances. These events give you a false belief within you that echoes, 'I am not enough'. You begin to disassociate from parts of yourself, and in doing so, you splinter your own identity like a mirror because your needs are not met in those moments.

Think of a scene when one of your caregivers or a teacher dismissed your feelings, ridiculed you, or made fun of you. You had to make sense of the outside world but were young and had little experience of life. In that moment, you did not feel loved or nurtured. There is only one way you could have interpreted it. The only conclusion you could come to was 'I am not loveable'. You did not have the ability to see the situation objectively. You were unable to understand that the other person was unable to meet your needs at that time because of their own internal issues. Perhaps they were too busy thinking about their own needs, or maybe they did not love themselves and, therefore, had not got the love inside themselves to give to you.

These narratives might stem from moments as fleeting as an unkind word from a teacher or an insensitive gesture from a loved one. Yet, their impact resonated deeply whether it was mental, emotional, physical abuse or more covert trauma. My dedicated approach to healing focuses on your traumas, which means that no trauma is small or insignificant when it comes to your emotional and physical wellbeing. They all impact you significantly but are buried within your subconscious mind, and you are, therefore, unaware of what you are holding on to emotionally.

Trauma is any situation or event that gives you a negative opinion of yourself. When you understand that, you can see that everyone has experienced hundreds of events that negatively affected them. People think trauma is what happens to you such as a divorce or car accident, these events are traumatic for sure. Trauma is what happens inside of you.

You were born completely dependent on other people to meet your needs, feed you, change you when you were soiled, and protect you. You had to trust that your caregivers and other adults around you would take care of you.

If they hurt you, beat you, degraded you, sexually assaulted or abused you or did not meet your needs in other ways, a whole range of emotions would have come up within you, such as emptiness, worthlessness, unimportance, insignificance, feeling betrayed, powerless, helpless, angry or enraged. All of this was too much to process and understand, so you had to suppress your feelings. But there is no escaping them, and these suppressed emotions show up in a variety of ways such as being quick-tempered, panic attacks, addictions, phobia, eating disorders, anxiety, depression and other long-term health issues. These feelings will always come out in a dysfunctional way, attracting your attention and asking you to do something about it.

Below are three scenarios or events I think you can relate to. They aren't what readily comes to mind when we think of trauma. These events haven't happened to any one person I have worked with, but I want you to imagine that they did in this example. When I work with clients, I regress them back to the events that caused the presenting issues. I want you to imagine the impact these would have had on you if you put yourself in that situation, how they would have affected your confidence and your self-esteem, and how the suppressed emotions could have become physical conditions.

**Fictional Client Scenarios:**

Just imagine that you are at your old primary school having a photograph taken because you were involved in a project there and the school wanted to reward the students with certificates and prizes. You left that school a few months ago and now attend a new one. You were quite excited about going back and seeing your old school friends. That vivid daydream did not match up to the reality that unfolded. Those cherished old school friends moved on, and they found new companions; they laughed with faces you did not recognise. It is this unexpected feeling of being alone, abandoned even, that fed into the seeds of doubt in your young heart. Suddenly, the world feels larger and colder, and you feel smaller and more alone within it, with thoughts of 'I don't matter. I don't belong. I'm not important' forming in your subconscious mind.

Picture another time when you were in your bedroom, and you overheard a conversation your parents were having. They were close enough for you to overhear their conversation, although they were unaware that you were listening. They were talking about your older sibling. They were speaking about them in a disapproving way. They weren't happy with the life choices they were making, and you did not like the way your parents were speaking about them. Hearing their words, you unconsciously decided that you were going to be a really good child, you were going to make your parents proud of you no matter what it took. In that moment, so many things occurred in your subconscious mind, although at the time, you were completely unaware. You created an invisible glass box crafted by concern and misunderstanding, keeping you from stepping too far astray, limiting the possibilities of who you could become. This box, though unseen, became a fortress, silently stipulating the terms of love and acceptance.

From this memory stems the underlying fear that followed you like a shadow: the fear of disappointing, leading to the potential loss of love of your parents, or worse, abandonment, all shaped by a conversation that was never even about you.

A few years later, you're at a party with your long-term partner, who you are totally in love with and believe is your forever love. You were with the person you cherished most in the world. The party was lively, an eruption of laughter and chatter echoed around the room.

As the evening wore on, you noticed that your partner was missing and nowhere in sight. Unease began to clutch at your heart. You made your excuses and went to go and find them, only to discover them kissing and flirting with someone else in the shadows of the garden. The moonlight cast a soft glow over your partner's lips and someone else's in a dance that was meant to be exclusively yours. You felt completely betrayed and shocked. Your whole world felt like it had unravelled before your eyes. You went back into the house, wrestling with the hurricane of emotions, shock, betrayal, and anger all swirling like a tornado inside of you.

You decide to think about the best action to take as fear clutches your heart. Later, you decide to do nothing and pretend the situation never happened. You effectively sweep it under the carpet in a desperate attempt to save your relationship.

In those turbulent moments, you made a choice. A choice to shroud yourself in silence, in the hope of clutching onto the fragments of love and the relationship you had built. You decided to pretend that the heartbreaking scene you witnessed was nothing but a phantom of the night.

However, suppressed emotions are like ghosts; they haunt. They linger in every interaction, seeping into the crevices of trust and entwining themselves around the pillars of your self-worth. Though your relationship continued, the connection you shared was filtered through a lens of silent withdrawal as protection, so you didn't get hurt again.

The agony didn't dissipate. It just wore different masks, morphing into anxiety and likely aching joints because it is a physical manifestation of emotional immobility.

Unacknowledged pain doesn't fade, it festers. It corrodes the very foundation of your being, undermining self-confidence, self-belief, and self-trust. Not all damage is visible, and not all wounds bleed.

In the end, trauma shapes you in ways you cannot foresee. Its effects are not just emotional or psychological but become integral to your physiology, embedding within you a chronic echo of the original hurt. Until you face these shadows, until you acknowledge and release these suppressed emotions, you will remain haunted by the echoes of the past. Emotional and physical pain are the same, they are roots from the same source.

When exploring the impact of past events on an individual's present psychological state, it's crucial to understand the profound effects that such experiences have on your beliefs, confidence, self-esteem, and even your physical health. To illustrate this, let us consider these scenarios:

**Childhood Bullying**:

Imagine a child experiencing relentless bullying at school. Peers taunt and exclude the child, leading to a deep-seated belief that they are unworthy or unlikable. This unrelenting negative feedback loop corrodes the child's confidence and self-esteem, which continues into adulthood. Such distressing experiences can manifest as anxiety, social withdrawal, or debilitating fears that hinder personal growth and development.

**Parental Neglect:**

Think of a scenario where a young person grows up in an environment of neglect. The lack of positive reinforcement, guidance, or emotional support from parents or caregivers is likely to give a child a sense of abandonment and a belief that they are undeserving of attention, care and love. These feelings give lack of self-worth issues and feelings and beliefs about being unlovable, which in turn impacts their ability to build healthy relationships and leads to emotional detachment. Physical symptoms, such as stress-related ailments, can absolutely arise from these emotional states, showing just how intertwined our emotional and physical well-being are.

From these examples I hope you can start to see that the damage isn't necessarily from what happened to you but the internal way it was processed and the conclusions you came to about yourself. In these pages I will help you alchemise that pain you felt into self love. It is seeing the truth behind the stories you created, so that you can see that it wasn't your fault. You were behaving in an age appropriate way. The other person or people involved had their own internal issues which were making them behave the way they did.

**Traumatic Loss:**

Consider a person who has suffered a sudden and traumatic loss of a loved one. The shock and grief may result in an internalised belief that the world is inherently unsafe, and that any happiness can be snatched away. This belief system can trigger extreme protective mechanisms within the person, such as fear of forming new attachments or emotional numbness, to avoid future pain. Physically, the suppressed emotions can lead to conditions such as insomnia, chronic tension, and other stress-related disorders.

By using regression therapy, I help clients revisit these impactful scenes to review them (not relive them) so that you can not only cognitively review and understand the source, but emotionally process and release the pent-up feelings associated with them. This cathartic process aims to recalibrate your current belief systems, restore self-esteem and confidence, and ultimately release the suppressed emotions that manifested as physical conditions, so much so that the physical symptoms can and do disappear. You then have a much more increased sense of self-worth, self-belief, self-trust, self-confidence, and self-love.

I offer my clients a non-judgmental safe space where you feel heard and valued, so that it is very safe for you to understand, release, and empower yourself from the things that hurt you. It allows you to come home to your true soul essence of who you really are and feel empowered to live your life of hopes and dreams on your own terms with joy and happiness in your heart.

# *Three Core Beliefs That Wound Us*

Core beliefs are the thoughts, assumptions, or conclusions you hold about yourself. These are deep-seated beliefs that are embedded in your subconscious mind and so often go unrecognised as they are below your conscious awareness. However, they constantly affect your life and deeply impact you. Rather like a computer program, these beliefs are running in the background and influence every decision you make. Your beliefs are formed by your experiences around you. As we discussed earlier, you can start to see how the traumatic events that you encountered negatively affect how you feel about yourself at a deep level.

Let's simplify core beliefs into just two that truly wound and impact us:

*I don't belong/I can't connect to other people.*

*What I want is unavailable to me.*

These two beliefs feed down into the ultimate wound which is 'I am not enough'. You can add any adjective you want into that sentence such as:

*I am not smart enough, I am not good enough, I am not kind enough and I am not loveable enough.*

Can you see how significant these core beliefs are?

The 'I am not enough' wound made you separate part of yourself from the rest of you, like a splintered piece of glass. This separation of yourself means you have fragmented your energy; you detached from yourself, which means that you love yourself less. Lack of self-love is the ultimate root cause of depression, anxiety and other long-term physical diseases and illnesses.

Healing allows you to return to that oneness, the soul essence of who you truly are. That is real self-love. Self-love isn't really an emotion, but more a state of being. Self-love allows you to connect to the truth of who you really are, your soul essence. But here's the vibrant truth, a declaration I am going to shout to you from the mountain tops:

## YOU ARE ENOUGH

## YOU ARE WORTHY

## YOU ARE LOVE

Every piece, every fragment, every shard of your being is worthy of love, especially your own.

The real truth is that you are an amazing, extraordinary, incredible being. The word 'enough' does not even fit into that sentence because you are so much more.. You are a diamond shimmering in the dark, illuminating the universe with your energy and light.

The self-love journey is not about discovering something new but more about a tender reunion with the parts of yourself you thought you had lost. It's about mending the fractures and polishing your internal mirror until you can see yourself clearly, brilliantly, and fully.

Recognising that self-love isn't just a part of your well-being, it's a foundation for your mental, physical, social, intellectual, financial and spiritual health. When you have a lack of self-love, it can snowball into the darkness that clouds your days with depression or anxiety and burdens your body with illness. By confronting these thought patterns with the ability of a warrior and the gentleness of a caregiver, we can begin to rewrite the story together. We will talk about this in more detail later with real tips and techniques to help you.

Trauma causes you to disassociate from yourself; reconnection is healing. Later in the book, I will help you reconnect to yourself.

*Healing at your personal root cause is the master padlock and the real master key is self-love.*

# The A-Z of Ailments, Diseases and Symptoms

A s we discussed earlier, every time you think a thought, your body generates an emotional response as well. Your body speaks the truth, and its language is pain and symptoms. Where the symptoms are in your body tells a deeper story. Not every symptom will be listed here, but you will begin to understand what is happening.

Your body is so literal with its messages. Pain and symptoms on the right side of your body are about the current time, the right here, right now moment. Pain and symptoms on the left side are about issues in your past. Where the symptoms occur gives a deeper story and a bigger picture of what is happening within you.

In this chapter, I will discuss various ailments and illnesses and enlighten you with information about what each of these can signify for you. This list is not exhaustive but covers most ailments/illnesses so you can interpret and decode what your body is saying to you.

## Accidents

Even what appear to be accidents are your subconscious and body's way of conveying messages. Whatever part of the body is affected gives a deeper meaning. All accidents show a tension you feel or inner conflict you are unable to communicate. No accident happens for no reason. A vehicle or mode of transport is an extension of your consciousness.

## Acne

Acne is like a distress signal asking you to acknowledge and release your inner turmoil and pain. My clients have taught me that their skin afflictions speak of a profound emotional struggle, a plea for recognition and understanding. 'Will someone please notice the pain I am in?' 'I am uncomfortable in my own skin'. These are the silent thoughts behind every blemish and breakout.

It's no coincidence that acne tends to mar your face, the mask you present to the outside world. This mask, when blemished by acne, broadcasts your deepest insecurities for all to see. Your skin is showing your feelings of inadequacy, manifesting visually, a representation of your hidden fears.

The irony of acne is that it amplifies the insecurities it stems from. We live in a universe that mirrors your beliefs back to you, and so your anxieties about worthiness become self-fulfilling, giving rise to further acne which, in turn, heightens your self-consciousness. It's a cruel cycle, one that seems relentless and insurmountable.

I speak from experience, having battled acne from my

teenage years well into my 30s. I remember the feelings of vulnerability, how it felt like walking about with an open wound for everyone to see. No cream or treatment offered lasting relief because they only served as a temporary veil over a much deeper issue. What I had not understood then was the influence of suppressed emotions, an unseen force dictating the state of my skin.

Skin conditions, I've come to understand, are physical manifestations of emotional scars. It wasn't until I addressed the suppressed wounds, the stored-up sentiments of not being good enough, that real healing began.

Now, as I reflect on the years of skin struggles, I wish I had known how deeply our psyche and skin are intertwined. That awareness could have led me to seek not just topical solutions but emotional resolutions. But perhaps my long fight with acne was necessary to bring me this knowledge, a wisdom I can now share with others to help them on their paths to healing.

Acne is a teacher, although a harsh one. It pushes you to confront the parts of yourself you would rather keep hidden and ultimately guides you toward a path of self-discovery and acceptance. Once you learn to address the underlying emotional challenges, to peel away the layers of self-doubt, you may find that your skin and your sense of self clear, as if a veil has lifted, revealing the beauty of your authentic self to the world.

## Addiction

An addiction to anything, whether food, alcohol, drugs, shopping, sex, gambling, etc, is a way to self-soothe and fill the empty void within yourself with something external to make you feel better. The problem is that until the emotional reason for the addiction has been addressed, the pattern is likely to keep repeating. All forms of addiction are a means of trying to find something that fills the void within you. The void within is a lack of self-love and connection, caused and created through trauma that made you disassociate from yourself or even self-loathe. There's a wounded child behind the addiction. It honestly breaks my heart that we have made drugs illegal, which then brings more shame onto an addict, which creates more wounds within the already emotionally traumatised person. I am not saying that drugs should be legalised, that is a completely different topic and not one for today. What I am saying is that the shame we have around the subject of addiction sends more deep loathing into the already emotionally wounded and already traumatised person.

It becomes clear, then, that the battle against addiction is not just about curbing a physical dependency but about healing deep-seated emotional wounds. The framework surrounding substance abuse, such as the illegality of drugs, inadvertently compounds shame upon those already scarred by trauma, escalating the cycle of addiction rather than nurturing the recovery that could blossom from compassion and understanding. There lies the profound change, not in the substance or behaviour itself, but in addressing the underlying emotional reasons powering the addiction cycle. By acknowledging and nurturing the wounded child within, you pave the way for true healing and transformation.

## Adenoids

The adenoids swell when a child does not understand the adult world. It may reflect the tension in their family as they may feel less significant and perhaps in the way. Removing the adenoids does not address the emotional root cause.

## Allergies

Allergies are the body's misguided immune response to harmless substances. The clients I have worked with all began from past life dramas with similar emotional links to this life. Any allergy is a way of protecting yourself from the outside world.

Deep-seated memories and past traumas can manifest in this current lifetime as a protective mechanism and a way to shield yourself from perceived threats based on previous encounters.

For instance, individuals with an allergy to pollen might subconsciously associate this with a threat from nature due to traumatic events in a past life, perhaps as a healer or 'medicine person' who met an untimely demise. In this understanding, the allergy is a barrier, preventing the individual from engaging closely with nature to avoid repeating past perils.

Similarly, allergies to domestic animals might arise from past life experiences where an animal, initially perceived as friendly or rescuing, betrayed that trust by leading the individual to danger or even death. The resulting allergy acts as an unconscious deterrent, keeping these animals at bay to prevent re-experiencing the trauma.

Such interpretations of allergies emphasise the importance of holistic healing that accounts not only for the physical manifestation but also for the emotional, psychological, and spiritual dimensions. They can help to dissolve the 'invisible shield' of allergies and promote harmonious living without the fear of past life traumas.

## Alopecia

Hair represents power, so hair loss represents powerlessness, a loss of connection with yourself and the outside world. Hair loss can indicate you are trying to control everything and are not trusting the flow of life. Whether you are experiencing patchy hair loss or baldness, the tension within is much the same.

## Alzheimer's Disease

An Alzheimer's patient often feels despair, isolated and

abandoned. Before becoming ill, they often attempt to control their life and others around them, They often have a lack of sense of direction and lack of memory to avoid their reality.

## Ankles

Issues with the ankle is the body's way of conveying to you that you are feeling inflexible in moving forward in life. The left ankle denotes something in the past you are unable to move forward from, and your right is about the current time. If both ankles are affected, it means there is something in the past and present that is causing you issues. Any issue with your bones is about feeling undervalued.

## Anorexia

Fear of being yourself, fear of taking space in the world, fear of growing up, needing to disappear because the feeling of the joy of living has left you.

## Anus

Holding on to issues and wanting to control situations. 'What is a pain in the bum to you?' Your body is so literal in its messages. I worked with a client once, and she said, 'That's a pain in the bum' all the time, and that was exactly where her pain was. Be careful of the language you use because our words cast spells, which is why it is called spelling.

## Anxiety

The subconscious mind is void of a timeline, so it fails to distinguish between yesterday, today, and tomorrow and can only acknowledge the ceaseless 'now moment'. The younger, more vulnerable version of you has yet to realise that you have blossomed into an adult and are, therefore, much more capable than you were as a dependent child. There is still a little child within you that feels scared and unhealed, and that wounded part of you contributes to your emotional state now. Recognising this internal process becomes the first step towards soothing the anxious impulses that arise. Your subconscious mind is hardwired to keep you safe and what better way than to keep you on high alert? The words you tell yourself and the pictures you form in your head influence your thoughts and reactions in your body, so be mindful of what you are telling it. Your mind can only get an understanding of what is going on externally by your thoughts, emotions and reactions. Feeling excited and feeling anxious are very closely related, so tell yourself you are feeling excited, and you will start to feel calmer.

Healing the emotional root cause of anxiety is key to having a calm and focused mind. Remember, your subconscious mind is 95% of your mind, and its language is emotion, so emotion over logic will almost always win. The subconscious mind is triggered by emotion rather than the event that is occurring.

## Arms

Issues with your arms are about holding on to things emotionally that you need to let go of. Your elbows are your love joints, as this is how you embrace your loved ones. Depending on which side of the body you are experiencing pain and symptoms tells you if it is from an issue in the past or present situation.

## Arthritis

In general, arthritis is a feeling of being undervalued and unable to move forward in life. Joints give us mobility, so issues with your joints show the inflexibility you feel in moving forward in life. Your arms are about holding on to things emotionally, and your legs and hips are about not being able to move forward in life. Arthritis is usually linked to close relationships that made you feel restricted and undervalued in the past, and sometimes, these relationships are still ongoing.

## Asthma

The feeling of being stifled or constricted by the outside world. The asthma issues I have worked with have had links to a death in a past life. It is the emotional connection to the past life, rather than the event itself that had similar emotional ties to how the client was feeling this lifetime when the symptoms began.

## Autoimmune Disease

Autoimmune disease is the body attacking itself. People

with autoimmune issues feel attacked, are unsure of how to defend themselves, and feel disconnected from themselves and others. Where the symptoms are gives a deeper understanding and clarity to what is happening emotionally behind the presenting issues.


## Back problems

Your back and spine are about not feeling supported and carrying an emotionally heavy load.


## Balance – lack of balance

Feeling like you are on shaky, unstable ground emotionally. You don't feel stable with yourself and your life.


## Bladder

The bladder and kidneys eliminate toxins from the body. The predominant emotion is fear and potentially feeling in danger, fear of letting go or holding on to people or situations. The need to urinate may also be used as a means of escape.


## Blood

Blood is the life source, so any issues with blood are related to a feeling of a lack of joy or a sense of purpose and fulfilment. Bleeding is a fear of your own life force, feeling out of control.

## Boils

This person feels anger but is unable to express it. The location of the boils on the body tells a deeper story of the emotional link or tie.

## Bones

Feeling stuck, undervalued, and unable to move forward in life and feeling unable to make the current decisions. The affected bones give a deeper understanding of the emotional issues.

## Bowel

The bowel allows us to eliminate waste, so any issues are often around fear of letting go (constipation) which is often related to close relationships, or trying to flush out a toxic situation or toxic relationship (diarrhoea).

## Brain

Your brain is your control centre. It sends and receives messages to and from your body to make sense of your internal and external world. Any issues are about not receiving messages or not acting on them. There can be a fear of having to control everything rather than allowing life to flow.

## Breasts

Breasts are how we nurture infants, so any issues are about being unable to nurture yourself or not being able to nurture others in the way you desire. Cancer has the predominant emotion of anger, so there's repressed anger around being unable to nurture or not feeling nurtured.

## Bruising

Bruising easily denotes not focusing enough attention to yourself and your own needs. Perhaps you feel the need to control others, and not allowing yourself the freedom you need. Where the bruising occurs on your body gives a deeper picture of what is going on.

## Bulimia

When we are very young, food is one of the only things we have some control over. Food is a way of filling the void. What is missing is love.

## Cancer

There is a message behind cancer that you need to understand so that the root cause can be released. It tells you there is something significant that you need to change so that you can release your internal suffering. The way cancer presents itself gives a deeper story of what is happening internally. The predominant emotion behind cancer is repressed anger, anger that, because it is suppressed, is turned inwards.

## Chronic conditions

You are not meant to be living with chronic conditions. It just means you have not fully understood the messages behind it and let go of the suppressed emotions that are keeping it there.

## Chronic fatigue

This is the subconscious trying to offer you protection from the pain you have endured emotionally and physically, trying to offer you a way of going within and being with yourself, to escape your current situation, to lock you away and protect yourself, almost like a blanket.

## Colds

Feeling sorry for yourself and the need to take time out. There is often an emotional issue going on with someone you are close to, at work or home. Anything to do with the lungs is how you interact with the outside world, so you feel restricted and are putting extra pressure on yourself.

## Constipation

Constipation shows an unwillingness to let go of things emotionally. You have to keep it all in. What are you not letting go of that you perhaps need to?

## Cough

Anything related to your throat has to do with your voice, so it is about words you need to say becoming stuck in your throat, causing irritation.

## Crohn's disease

It usually occurs in a person who is keen to get approval from someone who is close to them at the expense of their own needs. Pushing your own emotional needs down to meet other people's needs and losing yourself and your identity in the process.

## Deafness/hard of hearing

We subconsciously turn off hearing to things we don't want to hear. You may feel trapped in a relationship and not feel you can escape. Apart from being about issues with hearing others, it can also be about not hearing your own internal guidance.

## Depression

Depression is about de-pressing your emotions; you have learnt to press or push your emotions down. Depression creates the feeling of being isolated, and not wanting to face life. It is chronic sadness. Depression often has roots in childhood, where your child-self felt lost, abandoned, unloved, and sometimes replaced. These wounds cut deep. It made you feel unlovable, unable to connect to yourself or others, fearing abandonment and rejection, so you subconsciously locked yourself away. This unhappy depression is like a blanket that doesn't offer much security but perhaps stops society from rejecting you again because you withdrew into yourself first.

## Diabetes

There is a lack of joy, sweetness, and love of life. It is important for you to reconnect and love yourself.

## Disease

Disease is dis-ease, it is a disconnection within. Your body loves you and is giving you messages telling you there are unhealed parts within that need to be brought back into balance. It is less about curing and more about bringing you back into feeling whole and complete. Symptoms are like warning lights on a vehicle's dashboard alerting you that there is something internal that needs addressing. Once the suppressed emotions lying behind the symptoms have been addressed and released, the symptoms can and do disappear.

## Dizziness

Feeling unstable, insecure in your life, not rooted and on shaky ground emotionally.

## Ears

Ear issues are about not wanting to hear what others are saying or not listening or hearing your own internal guidance and messages.

## Eczema

The skin is the biggest organ of the body. Skin issues are your body's way of attracting attention to the outside world. 'Will someone take notice of the pain I am in, that I am unable to verbally express', or 'I am feeling uncomfortable in my own skin'. Where the eczema is on your body will give you clues about what it relates to emotionally.

## Elbow issues

The elbow is the love joint; it is how you embrace others. It is about feeling inflexible or rigid and not being able to let go of people or circumstances you need to, and it is often related to people close to us. Any issues with bones are about feeling undervalued, so you feel undervalued in loving relationships.

## Erectile dysfunction

The male reproductive organs represent a man's masculinity. They are also situated along the meridian line of the body, which is about feeling powerful. Think of the meridian line going down your body in the same place as your spine. So, there are no surprises then, that any issues along this line are about feeling powerless. This issue can be caused by toxic relationships where the man feels powerless, a victim or has feelings of guilt around sex or a sexual encounter.

## Emphysema

Feeling restricted, fear of life. A chapter ends in life perhaps, and the new chapter opening may feel sad or uninspiring. My great-uncle developed this after his wife died. I was a child then. Understanding what his body was saying back then makes so much sense to me now.

## Endometriosis

Feeling unable to be in our feminine energy, or express our feminine side and not feeling creative. Holding on to grief and guilt with loved ones.

## Eyes

Inability to see the situation as it is. A farsighted person is anxious and fears danger coming up from the future, the fear of change. Near-sighted people live in fear, fear of being caught without warning. I am nearsighted and currently working on improving my sight. It is so interesting to me that my parents argued a lot and there was often long, frosted silences that lasted weeks, or heated arguments. I read a lot in my bedroom with my cat as company. It is really interesting to me that I had perfect eyesight to read, but blurred the outside world using the power of eyesight.


## Eyes – detached retina

Something horrible happened that is too bad to be seen. Your body is telling you you're trying hard not to see a situation and playing it over in your mind, or it keeps presenting itself in your reality. You're not acknowledging it, so the emotions and fear stay in your body.


## Eyes – dry

You learned to shut your emotions down and literally turn off the tears. You are holding on to lots of emotions including anger.


## Face

Your face is the mask you present to the outside world, so any issues are related to feeling disconnected from the outside world or a feeling of separation.


## Fainting

Feeling insecure and on unstable ground emotionally.

Fainting is a means of temporary escape or a feeling of not being able to face up to a situation.

## Fatigue

A way of escaping our reality, often because you feel you don't fit in with your family or society in general.

## Feet

Your feet are your roots and control the direction you move in. They allow us to connect to the earth. Any issues with our feet show difficulty moving forward in life.

## Fever

Fever is your body's way of telling you that something is making you burn up inside, often related to work, home or situations close to you.

## Fibroid tumours

The emotions behind fibroid tumours are grief and guilt. It can often be about the desire to have children or pregnancies that didn't go full term, although it can also be about unprocessed grief from family members passing.

## Fibromyalgia

The body is saying there is conflict within you. In my

experience, people suffering from this have often been through toxic relationships where it has been important to put the needs of others before their own, and it did not feel safe to share how they felt. These unexpressed emotions show up physically. Where the pain occurs in the body is giving you more of a message of what is going on.

Even though the person with these symptoms may have been through these kinds of relationships, it often stems from childhood because the relationship patterns experienced aren't random. The beliefs about yourself are formed when you are small, so it makes sense that the roots are formed there. Fibromyalgia can also be about unexpressed grief. Grief about the life you thought you were going to live, grief from losing loved ones when you were small and unable to process it because the adults around you were grieving and didn't know how to help you.

Chronic fatigue is the subconscious trying to offer you protection from the pain you have endured emotionally and physically, trying to offer you a way of going within and being with yourself, to escape your current situation, to lock you away and protect yourself.

**Fingers**

Fingers are used to connect with the world. You touch, hold objects and loved ones, write, play musical instruments, create things, and express yourself using your fingers and hands.

Your thumb is letting you know you are holding sadness, grief and loss. Your left thumb denotes something in the past and your right is an indication that it is something in the present moments that you need to let go of and release.

Your index finger is about holding on to self-blame, guilt and feeling undervalued.

Your middle finger is showing you that you are holding on to feelings of jealousy, envy, anger and feeling powerless.

Your ring finger is about love, so the pain and symptoms in this finger are about close relationships and people you are intimate with.

Your little finger is how you feel you show up in the world, your place in society, feeling undervalued.

Your left side is letting you know there are issues in the past this relates to, and your right side is saying there is something in your current, right here, right now moment.

## Flu

Your lungs are about how you interact with the outside world in the same way you give and take a breath. Flu brings to your awareness that you feel out of the flow of life, restricted, perhaps emotionally smothered. Lungs indicate a loss of joy and fulfilment. Flu is a way of making you rest.

## Food poisoning

Food poisoning is not random or an accident. There is a message behind this too. If a group suffers from it at the same time, it is because they are all feeling similar tensions within themselves. Ask yourself questions such as 'How did I feel before I ate?' or 'How did I feel around the people at the table?' Did you go to the restaurant willingly or did you feel obliged to go? Do you have a fear of losing everything? Answers to these questions will help you to understand what is going on behind the scenes.

## Fractures

The emotions behind fractures are feeling restricted, undervalued, a big tension within you. your body is telling you to take a different path.

## Gallstones

Gallstones are feelings of aggression, anger, and frustration that have been building up for some time and haven't been resolved.

## Gas pain

When you get trapped wind, it is because you are pushing your emotions down. There is tension in your body, a restriction between holding on and letting go, and a push-pull feeling that causes stress in your stomach.

## Gout

We are told that the body produces too much uric acid which causes sudden pain and swelling in our joints such as big toe, ankles and feet. When I worked with this issue it was about feeling restricted in moving forward with their plans in life, unable to see a different solution to the problem they were facing. Just the next day after working together, my client reported that the pain was gone as though it had never been there because the session brought up different solutions that were easier to carry out, so they felt less burdened and much more in control of their life.

## Haemorrhoids

Difficulty in letting go of emotions, situations, and people. What has become a pain in the butt in your life?

## Hair

If you think of a lion with its mane, you think of a very powerful animal. Hair represents power, so hair loss is powerlessness, a loss of connection with yourself and the outside world, and holding on to lots of tension and trauma.

## Hands

Hands are used to hold on to and let go of things. Any issues with hands are about holding on to things emotionally that need to be let go of. See 'Fingers' for additional insights.

## Hay fever

Many allergies are from past life traumas with an emotional connection to this life. Previous sessions have revealed that it wasn't safe to be in nature; it was perceived as dangerous in the previous life. So, the subconscious mind is trying to protect you from the perceived danger even though what happened in the past is unlikely to happen again.

## Headaches

Pressure from having to perform a certain way that feels false to you, not in alignment with yourself or your personal needs. It is often about masking your feelings.

## Hearing

You don't want to hear what others are saying or listen to your own internal guidance and messages. The right side is something in the present you don't want to hear, and the left side is about something from the past.

## Heart issues

Heart issues are about love and close relationships.

## Hernia

The tension within you is so much that your abdomen cannot contain it.

## Herpes

Herpes often occurs when a person is looking outside of themselves for love and feels shame and guilt around sexual relationships.

## Hips

Hip pain means struggling to move forward in life in your desired direction. This desire may be one you are unaware of consciously, so your subconscious mind is trying to move you forward in a certain direction that you aren't perhaps taking notice of.

## Hives

Hives occur when you are trying to take part in a family or community but feel irritated by them or the attitude of an individual or even the atmosphere that is being created there. It is telling you that something is getting under your skin.

## Hypothyroidism

The thyroid is in the neck near the larynx. The thyroid regulates your metabolism. Hypothyroidism alerts you that you have difficulty communicating and are unable to confront others. You feel that people misunderstand you and are frustrated. You are always busy and never stop. You felt misunderstood as a child or that no one attempted to understand you, so you gave up on yourself, and often don't trust your own opinions of a situation. What are you running away from? This is a great question to start seeing what lies underneath.

## Hyperthyroidism

The thyroid is the body's accelerator. Although the root causes of difficulty communicating or feeling heard when you do are the same as hypothyroidism, the difference is that you concluded that there is no point in running away and feel indifferent to the outside world.

## Immune system

When your immune system works well, you feel in harmony with the outside world and within yourself. People with autoimmune issues, allergies, and intolerances feel attacked, are unsure of how to defend themselves, and feel disconnected from themselves and others. Where the symptoms are gives a deeper understanding and clarity to what is going on.

## Impotence

Impotence is the incapacity of the male to have sex due to the inability to have an erection. The emotional root is about feeling powerless, a victim, shame and guilt. It can be for a variety of reasons such as fear of hurting his partner, or losing them emotionally, or because his partner has, or had, a health condition. He may have an underlying root of feeling like a victim perhaps because of narcissistic, abusive or toxic relationships. It can also stem from a past life where a vow of celibacy may have taken place, to give a few examples. See also erectile dysfunction.

## Incontinence

Incontinence comes from a feeling of loss of control over a situation or himself. Consider animals and how they urinate to mark their territory, it is much the same in urinary incontinence. It is an involuntary action to mark our territory. Bowel incontinence is often about feeling fearful and/or trying to flush out a toxic substance or situation.

## Indigestion

Stomach issues are your body's way of saying you are finding it difficult to express feelings or digest what is going on. What is the uncomfortable situation you are facing or were facing when the symptoms began?

## Infections

It is important to understand that it is more about what is going on in your mind rather than the outside source that caused the infection. Otherwise, everyone would have the same infections and symptoms. It is time to remind ourselves that our body doesn't lie and is always speaking to us in pain and symptoms. There is an inner conflict, anger at yourself, where the infection lies which will help uncover a deeper meaning to what the anger or conflict is about.

## Infertility

There can be so many reasons why a man or woman is infertile. There is conflict within the person, for a variety of reasons. For example, a woman may have a deep subconscious fear about being pregnant because her mind sees it as being bigger/fatter which she has tried to avoid being much of her life, or perhaps she has a more masculine career so being pregnant and her own identity with the outside world doesn't match, there is inner conflict. The subconscious mind will do whatever it can to avoid perceived danger, and it is run by emotional responses, not logical ones.

## Inflammation

Inflammation comes from the Latin word 'inflammare', which means 'set on fire'. Your body is saying you are on fire and have angry thoughts. Where the inflammation is in your body will give more meaning to what you are feeling 'on fire' or angry about.

## Influenza

See flu

## Insect bites

If you are regularly being bitten by insects, you are punishing yourself and feeling guilty about small things.

## Insomnia

Insomnia is the subconscious mind's way of keeping you on high alert. The reason usually stems from childhood. Remember, your subconscious mind doesn't understand the past, present and future, but only the current moment. It is doing its best to protect you. Healing at your unique root is key to allow you to sleep well again.

## Irritable Bowel Syndrome (IBS)

You are trying to seek approval from people close to you at the expense of losing yourself in the process. You have a deep-seated fear of being alone and of rejection.

## Itching

Something is getting under your skin emotionally and your body is telling you to move forward from it.

## Jaw issues

Anything about your mouth is about being unable to speak your truth and share how you feel. Jaw issues are saying you are holding on to a lot of tension, such as anger and frustration about not speaking up, or if you do, you don't feel heard.

## Joints

Joints give mobility, so any issues with your joints are about feeling restricted and inflexible. Which joint(s) is affected gives deeper meaning to what is going on.

## Kidney issues

Kidneys flush out toxins within your body. It is often about trying to flush a toxic situation or relationship away, there's a lot of fear in the body.

## Knees

Knees allow you to move forward, so there is resistance and inflexibility to moving forward; you are feeling restricted and undervalued in your ability to take the next step.

## Laryngitis

The larynx contains the vocal cords and functions as a voice box for producing sound. Laryngitis is about fear of speaking up, fear around what you have to say and how it will be received.

## Legs

Legs help you move forward. Issues with your legs mean there is resistance and tension in moving forward in life. Whether the issue is felt on the right, left, or both sides of the body gives more clarity about what the issue is about. Right side of the body is the right here, current moment and the left side denotes issues in the past.

## Leukaemia

Leukaemia is a type of blood cancer and has emotional roots in a lack of self-esteem, feeling undervalued and unable to take responsibility for yourself at a deep subconscious level.

## Ligaments

Ligaments connect two bones, so issues with them involve feeling inflexible and undervalued. Which ligaments are affected give deeper meaning to the emotional root.

## Liver

The liver is the largest internal organ. It filters blood, stores glycogen, and converts carbohydrates into fat. Issues with the liver are related to fear of scarcity, such as money and love, toxic situations, and difficult family members. Liver issues are often about suppressed anger.

## Lungs

Lungs allow you to give and receive breath. You inhale a breath into your body and exhale it out. Therefore, the lungs symbolise your interaction with the world and your relationships. Issues with your lungs are about feeling restricted, smothered, fear of dying, or fear of not really living the life you desire.

## Menopause

Menopause is a stage in a woman's life when she is reaching the end of the possibility of having children. The symptoms experienced have a large bearing on thoughts and beliefs about yourself. It is often about feeling invisible, replaced by a younger generation, not feeling worthy and therefore feeling undervalued.

Menopause is a natural process and not a disease, so should not manifest in symptoms. For example, hot flushes are about natural sexual desires that still need to be expressed and experienced.

## Menstruation

Painful menstruation can be felt in the abdomen, head, breasts, and legs. Painful periods tend to be felt in women who find it hard to be in their feminine energy and resistance to being in their creative feminine power, which can be passed down through the ancestral line.

## Migraine

A migraine is more than a headache and often has disturbed vision and can cause vomiting and diarrhoea. The sessions I have had with clients have usually been about past life traumas that have emotional links to the current life.

## Mouth issues

The mouth, teeth, and tongue are the start of the digestive system and are part of how you communicate. Issues with your mouth are about being unable to speak up or communicate how you feel.

## Multiple Sclerosis

MS affects the muscles and nerves and is a form of paralysis. Nerves represent communication. Your nerves are like telephone wires running up and down your body so that information can be received to and from the brain. MS symptoms alert you to the fact that you do not feel valued and are experiencing communication issues, not listening to your own intuition, and feeling restricted by outside views/perceptions of yourself.

## Muscles

Muscles allow movement and flexibility, so any issues with your muscles are related to feeling inflexible and unable to move forward. The muscles that are affected give a deeper meaning to what is being conveyed.

## Nasal drip

A nasal drip signifies the tears that you can't or don't cry with your eyes.

## Neck

You use your neck to look around and see things from different angles. Your body tells you that you are not seeing every angle of a situation or perspective. You need to look through a wider lens at the possibilities in front of you.

## Nervous breakdown

A person who has a mental breakdown is feeling overloaded and overwhelmed with stress and worry. It is usually because they have a strong desire not to let go of anything and need to take care of it all which ends up with them feeling isolated and depressed.

## Neuropathy

Any issue with our nerves is about communication, stress , and worry. It could be that you're finding it hard to communicate with people close to you, loved ones, or colleagues and/or that you are not listening to your own internal guidance.

## Nose

There is a saying about not seeing something right under your nose, and funnily enough, that is what a blocked nose, or sinusitis, indicates. It points to the fact that you, or someone close to you, is putting pressure on you. When I worked with this issue previously, it was about trying to be perfect in every area of life, which gave way to a belief that there is never enough time or resources. Once we shifted that perception, the symptoms stopped.

## Nose bleed

A spontaneous nosebleed, rather than being hit, signifies the feeling of being mistreated or ignored. It is about a loss of happiness and joy in life.

## Oesophagus

The oesophagus is part of your digestive system. Issues with this often include feeling very hurt about what someone said or did and being unable to digest or believe what happened. Cancer in this area is intense anger around this situation and that anger has turned inward on yourself as it has been unable to be fully expressed.

## Osteoporosis

Osteoporosis is where bones become fragile and weak, particularly in the back. There are intense feelings of feeling replaced, undervalued and particularly unsupported.

## Overweight

Weight issues are seldom really about food. There is a conflict within about not accepting yourself for who you truly are because of the traumas you have experienced. Weight issues may be masking feelings of abandonment, a belief that you need to be bigger to protect yourself, or a fear of loss. Your subconscious mind perceives loss as painful, so if you are trying to lose weight, you may find using different language, such as 'I am choosing to drop a dress size', more productive. Ultimately, food is filling the void, an empty feeling within you. The empty feeling is a lack of self-love.

## Pancreas

The pancreas produces insulin, which helps regulate blood sugar levels. If the pancreas isn't working correctly, there is an underlying feeling that you aren't loved enough and lack joy in life.

## Panic attacks

Panic attacks can be a frightening and overwhelming experience. While the exact triggers will vary from person to person, panic attacks are emotionally connected to your past.

The root cause can be traced back to a significant event or experience that left a deep imprint on your subconscious mind. Even if you don't consciously remember the initial trigger, your emotional memory will still hold onto that charge, ready to be activated by similar situations in the present. It will feel the same emotionally and not necessarily like the actual physical event itself.

## Paralysis

The area of the body affected by paralysis will give a deeper meaning to what is happening emotionally within. Fear and indecisiveness are preventing the person from moving forward.

## Parathyroid

See thyroid


## Parkinson's disease

The person with Parkinson's disease is likely to have been holding onto tension within themselves for some time around feeling agitated and frustrated. It's usually around feeling other people having control without being able to react to it as it didn't feel safe to share their feelings, so the tension within has been building up within themselves.


## Prostate

The underlying root of issues with the prostate is feeling inadequate and powerless.


## Psoriasis

Skin is the organ between you and the outside world. Skin issues are emotionally about putting up a barrier between you and the people around you, usually to protect you from getting emotionally hurt again. Look at my website to see some remarkable photos of skin healing. There are several photos of past clients before and after working with me. One client had a single session with me who had psoriasis over much of his body. The results within a 2-week window are quite remarkable. Take a look at my website for photos of clients' healing their skin.

https://wellnesswithrachel.co.uk/

## Psychosis

It is the ultimate way to separate ourselves from reality, family, and community. It is about trying to escape reality.

## Rash

There is an irritation, something getting 'under your skin' emotionally. Where the rash appears on your body will give more information about what is occurring emotionally.

## Raynaud's Disease

You are holding on to people and situations really tightly that you need to be letting go of.

## Reproductive organs

Problems with this system are because of the difficulty for women to embrace and accept their feminine power. Issues with men's reproductive organs are because of them not being able to embrace their masculinity. Reproductive organs are our creative centres, so not being in our creative energy can also cause issues.

## Rheumatoid Arthritis

This disease affects joints, so RA alerts you that you feel restricted in moving forward in life and are holding tightly to emotions, situations, or people that make you feel undervalued. You are holding on to things or situations that you need to let go of so that you can live a healthier life. The affected joints will give more clarity to the root cause.

## Scoliosis

Scoliosis is a curvature of the spine, so it is about feeling unsupported and not being able to stand up for yourself. Scoliosis occurs in puberty and is connected to the relationship the child has with their parents.

## Shoulders

Issues with shoulders are because you carry emotional burdens that aren't your own.

## Sinus problems

Sinus issues are about other people putting pressure on you, particularly those who are close to you, such as work colleagues or partners. Very often, it is you who is putting the most pressure on yourself. It is very interesting that I suffered from chronic inflamed sinuses for 4 years, which coincided with a toxic relationship I was in, even though it appeared to have started while I was swimming.

## Skeletal issues

Overall emotions of feeling restricted and undervalued.

## Skin

Skin is the biggest organ of the body and protects you from the outside world. 'Will someone please notice the emotional pain I am in?' 'I am uncomfortable in my own body'. Where the skin issue is located on your body, gives a deeper picture of what is going on internally. Take a look at my website for photos of clients' healing their skin the QR code or link will take you there.

https://wellnesswithrachel.co.uk/

## Slipping accident

The body is telling you that you are feeling emotionally on unstable or unsteady ground.

## Smell

Your sense of smell adds texture to the food you eat, and you gain more understanding of the world around you.

People with reduced or no sense of smell tend to fall into bed exhausted and are mentally busy during the day. The body is asking for more chances to relax and to avoid putting too much pressure on yourself.

## Sore throat

Words you need to say are getting stuck in your throat. What do you need to communicate?

## Spine

The spine forms the support system of your body. Issues with your spine are telling you that you feel unsupported and not able to stand up for yourself.

## Sprains

Sprains show that you are feeling restricted and inflexible. When you notice which joint is affected, you can start to understand the tension within.

## Stomach problems

When you suppress your emotions rather than process them, you can experience digestive problems. A great question to ask yourself to gain more clarity around the issue is, 'What am I not digesting or able to stomach?'

## Suicidal thoughts

I write these words with so much love and compassion for anyone feeling this way. By working with clients who have had suicidal thoughts, I have seen first-hand that there is a part within that feels so much emotional pain it is almost unbearable to live with. These thoughts and feelings weren't present from birth. They are learnt responses to the stories you told yourself from an early age; stories that were crafted to make sense of a world when your emotional needs went unmet. In these stories, you saw yourself as a flawed character. Then the beliefs of 'I am not lovable', 'I don't matter', and 'I am unworthy of love' become how you saw yourself. Your reality only served to reinforce these internal doubts, fears and self-loathing, which trapped you in a cycle of perceived rejection and abandonment and worse.

Recognising these beliefs for what they are, mere interpretations rather than absolute truths, is the first step towards rewriting your internal stories. This understanding is not just empowering; it's liberating. There is nothing wrong with you. You are made of love and are on the planet for a reason. It is possible to heal those hurts so that you can see yourself in the true light of who you really are, and it truly doesn't take long to achieve when you heal at the root.

## Tapeworms

A person who has worms feels unprotected and a victim.

## Teeth problems

Your teeth issues involve an inability to speak up, fear of sharing how you feel, and difficulty showing assertiveness.

## Thigh

Issues with your lower limbs mean you have difficulty moving forward in your life path.

## Throat issues

Fear of speaking up and fear of how your words land with others.

## Thyroid issues

Unable to speak up and needing to avoid confrontation - see also hyperthyroidism and hypothyroidism.

## Toes

With all joints, there are underlying emotions of inflexibility and rigidity in moving forward in life. Which foot is affected tells whether it relates to a past or present situation.

The right foot is about the right here and now, present moment, while the left is an issue in the past. Issues with your big toe indicate a lack of joy in life and a feeling that life is a big duty.

## Trachea

Also known as the windpipe, this area is letting you know that you are feeling restricted, suffocated with life.

## Ulcerative Colitis

This is a chronic inflammation of the bowel. A person who has UC has diarrhoea, pain, blood and mucus loss. A person who presents these symptoms has lost their identity, feels their family has rejected them, doesn't feel like they fit in, and their feelings don't matter.

## Ulcers

A person with ulcers is feeling other people are controlling their life.

## Urinary infections

Your body is telling you there is a toxic situation in your life that you need to remove or detach yourself from.

## Uterus

Issues with our uterus are about not feeling in your creative life force energy, not in your feminine power.

## Vagina

A vagina is part of the female reproductive organs, and issues here indicate that the female is not in her feminine energy.

## Varicose veins

Varicose veins are usually in the lower limbs, so your body is alerting you that you feel unable to move forward. As your veins carry blood to your heart, it indicates a lack of joy in life, being unable to express your emotions to the right person, and not feeling listened to or understood.

## Vertebrae

You are feeling tension, which is deeply rooted in not feeling supported or able to support yourself and feeling undervalued.

## Vertigo

You are not feeling centred or rooted in life, usually relating to issues at home, work or other close relationships.

## Vomiting

It represents the sick-to-the-stomach feeling you are experiencing in life. What are you not digesting or not able to accept?

**Wart/verruca**

You are feeling undervalued, trying hard to be perfect and feel frustrated because of the need to please people.

# Turning Pain to Passion

*Content warning: Rachel's story mentions toxic relationships, rape, abortion, suicidal thoughts and car accidents.*

I want to share my story so that you can perhaps see yourself in mine. My story may give you a deeper understanding of how your past has influenced your present in ways you perhaps haven't thought about before. The main reason for sharing my story is so that you can see what is possible for you when you heal and release the old stories and emotions that are perhaps keeping you in the same cycles and behaviours. Healing is possible, and it truly doesn't have to take countless sessions, or years to heal and release.

As a child, I was insecure and scared. I felt that everyone had a better understanding of life than I had. Later, I realised that even my birth story, which was recounted every year, had a big impact on my self-confidence. I was born by caesarean section. I was told that I 'didn't know the right way to be born', and that gave me a deep sense of shame and a belief that I shouldn't be alive because if I didn't know how to be born correctly, who was I to be on the planet? I felt like a fraud, and it was a secret I didn't want anyone outside of our family to discover. It seems almost laughable now, but as a child, I felt like an imposter, like I carried a big shameful secret that I really shouldn't be here and that no-one could find out in case I got whisked away somewhere scary and wouldn't be able to find my way home again. It truly felt like that big of a deal.

I was an anxious child at school. We often witnessed pupils getting the slipper on a Friday afternoon at primary school, so I lived in fear of that being me too, even though it was usually boys that received the punishment. Life generally didn't feel safe.

I grew up in a small village in England, before the invention of the internet. There was no library in the village, and the TV had only three channels initially, so my view of the outside world was limited, and I often felt isolated.

When I was small, I loved helping Dad cut our lawn. I had a toy lawnmower and sometimes I was allowed to hold the handlebars of my Dad's lawnmower with him which made me feel helpful. Mum spent endless hours teaching me how to skip using a skipping rope and Dad helped me learn to ride a bike. I loved my bike and spent many hours riding it through the countryside. It gave me a wonderful sense of freedom.

I was always looking for people to validate me and my opinions. It didn't feel safe to share who my favourite pop group was at school in case I gave a 'wrong' or unpopular opinion. I let my friends read my diaries and I didn't see anything wrong with that because I was seeking validation from them. I spent too much of my youth feeling anxious, insecure and afraid of everything.

When I was 19, I agreed to go on a date with a guy a friend suggested I go out with. So, again, buying into the idea that everyone else knew what was best for me, I went along with it.

I can remember exactly what I was wearing that evening. I was looking forward to going out to a local highly-recommended restaurant. I was wearing a dress with an autumn-shade leaf pattern, with a mandarin collar, buttoned to the neck, belted at the waist and mid-calf length. When I arrived at his parents' home, he told me to wait in the lounge. I sat on the edge of the sofa waiting for him. He eventually came into the room. I assume that we must have been completely alone in the house as he grabbed me in one quick movement and pushed me aggressively to the floor. He lifted my dress up and forced himself into me. I will never forget that animalistic look in his eye. His eyes looked dangerous. I felt sick. I just wanted it over. I felt powerless and hopeless and terrified. I dare not fight him; it didn't feel like a safe option. As suddenly as it began, it was all over, and he pushed me out of the front door. I felt so dirty, so humiliated, lost and deceived.

But worse was yet to come. I missed my next period. I was pregnant from being raped. The thought of having to tell someone what happened to me made me feel sick, anxious, terrified, humiliated and very ashamed. I decided to deal with it myself and booked a doctor's appointment. However, my dad saw me leaving the surgery and my mum confronted me. Her reaction was devastating. She immediately said that I must have done something to provoke the rape. Not being believed by my own mother was an extra wound of self-loathing and humiliation. I replayed that scene over and over in my head on a loop, but I really hadn't done anything to provoke the attack. I hadn't done or said anything. I hadn't even had the voice to stop him.

I had an abortion in a private hospital. Mum said that I needed to pay for it financially and emotionally then it wouldn't happen again as I needed to learn the lesson. It cut deeper than any knife could. But I vowed to myself that this experience wouldn't define me. I locked it in a box in my head, padlocked it, determined never to uncover it again. I thought I had dealt with it by locking it away. I had no clue then that this experience had lowered my sense of self-worth, self-belief, self-trust and self-confidence even more and increased my self-loathing so much that it actually impacted everything in my life.

I wrote my car off a few months later on my way to work. I really wasn't that bothered about what happened to me. It was a scary thing coming off the road on that freezing cold morning. My car was out of control on the extremely slippery bends on the icy back road and then it left the road and went towards a dyke in a field. Time seemed to go very slowly as the car rolled over onto its roof and bounced back on the road again, miraculously landing on all four wheels. Blood was pouring from the back of my head, and I had the urge to get out of the car in case it caught fire, but the doors wouldn't open, and I felt so tired I had to close my eyes. I was freezing cold and so very exhausted.

A lady in the house about half a mile up the road heard me scream as the car rolled and she called the ambulance. I was okay, I just needed half a dozen stitches in the back of my head.

After the accident, I promised myself I would take better care of me. It felt like I had been given a second chance at life. I bought a new ring a few weeks later as a visible promise to take better care of myself. I still wear that ring often now.

I fell in love in my late twenties and was so excited when he proposed. As soon as I said 'yes' to his proposal, I immediately told him that I had been raped and what happened that night. He said that he would have to rethink the proposal. It was a difficult conversation because it was the first time I had spoken to anyone about what had happened apart from my parents. I didn't blame him for feeling or saying he needed to think about it because I felt the same way. I felt like damaged goods.

That marriage lasted 14 years. We did have some good times and had children together.

In the last few months of being married to my husband, I had a dream about a childhood friend who had known me since I was small..

In the dream, my friend shook me, and I felt his breath on my face. It felt so real. He told me in the dream that I had to help him, and if I didn't, he would die. I sent him away three times in the dream, saying I couldn't help him because I was married and had a full life looking after my children and working. He came back each time insisting that I was the only one who could help him. I couldn't shake the dream; what if it held real meaning? I pondered on what to do for several days. I decided to reach out to him and send a text. I had his number stored on my phone, but hadn't contacted him in years. I knew I couldn't live with his death on my conscience. I knew that he was struggling and this impacted my decision.

I began to have contact with him daily by text to offer support at a difficult time in his life. I can't remember what the first text message was that I sent to him, but it was probably "Hi, how are you? Long time since we spoke, but I just thought you could do with a friend right now. You don't have to message back, but it would be good to hear from you". To my surprise, he did message me back and told me about a relationship he was in that wasn't helping his mental state.

We began texting daily. I remember saying I was his genie in his mobile phone and here to help support his mental state. Suddenly, five days passed, and I hadn't heard from him. I had a very uncomfortable feeling in the pit of my stomach that I couldn't shift. It was as though my body knew something was amiss. I tried calling him on his mobile every day during this texting silence, but my calls kept reaching his answerphone. Eventually, I managed to get hold of him.

To my surprise, he answered my call this time. But my relief of being in contact was quickly extinguished. He was at the side of a busy road waiting to walk in front of a lorry. It was such a difficult conversation as he wasn't making much sense because he'd been drinking and kept forgetting what I was trying to say to him, so I had to repeat myself constantly. The phone line connection wasn't great either. He said he felt lost and alone and there was no point in living anymore. I told him I loved him, and I would contact his parents and get the help he needed. At that time, I meant that I loved him like a brother I never had, human to human.

Fortunately, I was able to contact his parents and got them to be with him, support and comfort him. He came to live near me, as his parents had retired to a village nearby.

I felt somehow responsible for him because he didn't know anyone in the area. We often went for coffee together and I felt he leaned heavily on me emotionally. I moved out of my marital home, and it wasn't long before he moved in. Familiarity felt safe I suppose. We were both co-dependent for different reasons, although I didn't have that awareness at the time. Life was happy to begin with, but he soon became quick to give my children jobs around the house with immediate consequences if they weren't carried out straight away. We even had to ask for him to take things out of the garage because he had 'filed them away' and he said we would make a mess of things. What I failed to realise at the time was that full and empty bottles of alcohol were stored in the garage. It was like walking on eggshells trying hard not to put a foot wrong. He was very demanding, and I was always trying to keep the peace trying to create a 'perfect family' for me and the kids.

In 2016, I felt like the stuffing had been pulled from me again. It was a winter's day, nearing the end of the year and it felt like the end of everything I'd ever stood for, everything I'd ever worked for, and everything that got me up in the morning. It was as though my passion, my drive, my commitment had all been washed away. I felt broken; I'd never felt pain as raw as this before.

Trying to stay focused and continue as normal, I went upstairs to strip the bed. The pain inside was too much, and I sat down, tears cascading down my cheeks. I sobbed, I howled. The pain was so immense it felt physical. I felt like my heart had been ripped out, and perhaps it had if the sounds I was making were anything to go by.

I was crying because my two gorgeous children, who were, and still are, the centre of my world, had left to live with their father because they couldn't tolerate living with my partner and I any longer. He told me coldly that I needed to get over it, to move on and live my life. His reaction to my pain only made me feel worse.

I began to question my judgment and my actions; to really explore how I was feeling. How had I gotten to this point? He had promised me so much and now my future was in tatters before it had really begun. The reality was that he was denying the role that he played in my children leaving. I, on the other hand, understood my role in this heartbreaking decision that they had made. They were honest about why they couldn't live with us anymore and I knew my choices had led to this situation.

Everything had been great in the early days but he became demanding, setting tough rules for the kids, saying it was because I was 'too soft'. He would demand homework and other tasks to be done or started instantly. It was his way or the highway, there was no negotiating. And yet he refused to see or admit how he had a shared responsibility in their leaving. My children no longer being an active part of my everyday life was a huge shock. They were my main focus. I'd even taken a job at a local school so that I was at home when they got home from school and had school holidays together. Now I had to find my 'why' again; figure out what I was going to do to help distract myself from the emotional pain I was in.

So, here I am sitting on the bed, feeling destroyed, wondering how I got here when all I really wanted to do was to please people and make their lives happy.

Shortly after sitting on the bed and feeling like my life was over, a friend from school, Penny Francis, popped back into my life as though she knew I needed her. She is a spiritual medium and I owe so much to this wonderful lady. We spent the weekend together with another friend, Kate, discussing things. At the end of the weekend, I had formed some kind of plan; I intended to investigate finding a course locally to train to be a counsellor. I found one and started a course that had hypnotherapy training in the first year and counselling in the following two years. Hypnotherapy didn't interest me, or so I thought, but it was the best course I could find close to home. It turned out I wanted to learn more than the course provided, so I found an advanced hypnotherapy method and did both courses at the same time.

I was studying every hour I could, and I remember watching a training video during my lunch hour at work. I realised that I could have been in the therapy chair in the video because I had had similar toxic relationship issues and patterns throughout my life.

I had another wake-up call a couple of months later. I was involved in another car accident, a low-impact shunt this time, on my way to work. I knew my partner was at home in bed because I had just left the house, but when I tried calling him, he didn't answer. When I got home, I told him what happened, but he said I was making no sense. It was then that I realised he was drunk.

I sat down some time later and wrote two headings at the top of a piece of paper: 'Reasons to stay' and 'Reasons to leave'. The 'reasons to leave' column was much longer. There were only two things in the 'reasons to stay' column: He cooks and irons. I could do those things on my own.

I took legal advice, and I have never had anxiety like I experienced that year. Every day, the ache in my stomach and the feeling of breathlessness greeted me on waking, and it was there to tell me that today was another day to take action. The fear of staying where I was was much greater than the fear of the unknown.

I began to look for somewhere my children and I could live if they decided they wanted to be with me again. I had support from friends, but I had never felt so alone, like a little boat riding a never-ending tsunami wave, always feeling that I was about to capsize.

While my relationship was falling apart, I was renting a room in a local wellness centre and having amazing sessions with clients, including two with PTSD and psoriasis. Both of these issues were released in a single session. I was beginning to start believing in myself. I knew that I needed to get the message out there that the answers aren't outside of ourselves but in our own subconscious minds, and that life is for living and not therapy. More people need to know this and not feel stuck in a cycle of therapy for years and years.

I found the house I wanted to buy and found a buyer for our home too. I felt like I had been erased and a fragment of my former self. I was spent from over giving, constantly trying to please him trying to keep the peace and being his emotional punchbag. I didn't like myself very much, but I knew I was worth more than that.

There is someone else that needed to heal... me. It was to be my 50th birthday in a few months and the thought of dating again terrified me. The thought of being a single woman with just cats for company for the rest of my life was just as frightening. I didn't feel I could trust myself to date again, so I had a hypnotherapy session on why my personal boundaries were low and why I was a people pleaser. I won't go into detail of my session, but it came to light that as a child, I learnt that love was painful. So, as our subconscious minds have been built to do, it kept repeating situations and events that echoed that deep-seated belief in me that I was totally unaware of until now. After the session, I knew that the pattern had been broken for good for me. Moving out of our home and into my new space still took a lot of determination and I felt like giving up so many times.

I felt unsafe while I was living in our home, as I wasn't legally allowed to change the locks, and I was never sure if he would be coming back (he was no longer living there at this point). At the same time, I was still working through the process of healing from this relationship.

The day after my 50th birthday, I moved into my own home. I was determined to make the rest of my life some of the happiest times. My daughter moved back in with me, which gave me so much joy and eased my aching heart.

I did begin dating again to test my new ability to establish healthy boundaries and learn to trust myself again. I made a vision board of things I wanted in my life, including what qualities I wanted in the love of my life. I began to make a list: 'I want my man to be caring, considerate, tall, loving, kind....'.

The universe answered me; I joined two Stand In The Park groups during lockdown, and both gave me a link to a different group on Telegram. My new man was in both of these groups. Hurray for the law of attraction. I moved to the centre of England to be closer to him. It's funny, because Penny had told me in 2019 that I would move to the centre of England in a reading she did for me. I had no plans to do that back then and dismissed the idea. What is remarkable is that my boyfriend planted a tree to mark the centre of England when he was at primary school. Now, I live just a few miles away from that tree.

Just as we met, I decided to buy an inflatable hot tub. When I told my boyfriend about it he told me his story that he and his wife had bought a hot tub in lockdown, but she had become ill, and they decided to sell it without using it. She had promised him she would get him another just before she died, which was ten months before we met. I had seen a neighbour with an expensive one in their back garden and they spent more time working on the roof that covered it than being in it, so I was disinterested. I told my boyfriend how I felt and my sudden change of heart around it, and he got goosebumps. He believes that his wife was sending him a powerful message and had helped him to find me. The goosebumps and hot tub were his confirmation.

And here I am. The way I view myself has changed. I have gone from being co-dependent my whole life, to being independent. My unhealthy personal boundaries are healthier, and my self-belief, self-love, self-trust, and self-worth have also increased massively. I have also found my life purpose.

So much has changed in my life physically because my internal world changed. That is why I talk about this healing path as one of transformation and manifestation because when our internal thoughts change, our external world has to match.

The silver lining in my story is that I have turned my pain into my passion. Although it really didn't feel like it at the time, I am so glad that I went through this experience, as I have healed on a deeper level and released past trauma of rape and emotionally abusive relationships. My experience taught me so much more than any book could, about toxic relationships and I believe that has significantly helped me to be the outstanding therapist people consider me to be because I have been there on the other side and know first-hand how they make us feel.

Although the relationship with my boyfriend didn't stand the test of time, it was still proof that I have broken the pattern of toxic relationships. I am happy in my new environment. I have moved to a lovely area with plenty of beautiful scenery and so many exciting things to experience. I am looking forward to what the next chapter will bring.

*"The person leading you towards spiritual awakening is not the one who praised you or is nice to you. Your spirituality deepens because of those who insult you and give you a hard time. They*

*are your spiritual teachers in disguise" – Haemin Sunim.*

# *Unlock Your Wisdom To Heal – The Transformational Power of Self-Love*

In the previous chapters we have uncovered how trauma has a way of disconnecting you from yourself. It paved the way for harsh internal criticism, self-doubt, and, at its extreme, self-loathing. These feelings, however, aren't ones you were born with. They are learnt responses to the stories you told yourself from an early age, stories crafted to make sense of a world when your emotional needs went unmet. In these stories, you thought there was something wrong with yourself and the stories of 'I am not lovable', 'I don't matter', and 'I am unworthy of love', etc, were ones you told yourself on repeat. Then, external validation from the outside world only reinforced those internal doubts, trapping you in a cycle of perceived rejection and abandonment, shaping your perception of who you are and what you thought you deserve.

Here's the turning point, the moment of clarity. It is time to recognise these beliefs for what they are, mere interpretations of the outside world and not absolute truths about yourself. This is the first step towards rewriting your story. This understanding is not just empowering; it's liberating.

Remember your subconscious mind attracts what you believe at a deep subconscious level. Change your beliefs and your outside world shifts too.

The path to healing lies in embracing the simple yet profound truth that self-love is the antidote. It is the remedy that can mend the wounds inflicted by trauma, which causes illness and disease. By cultivating a deep love and appreciation for yourself, you start to reconstruct your shattered sense of self.

Self-love is not so much about indulgent self-care rituals or fleeting moments of pampering. It is about fundamentally shifting how you feel about yourself. It is about recognising your worth, embracing your flaws, and treating yourself with the same compassion and kindness you readily extend to others. It is loving your imperfectly perfect self.

As you embark on this path of self-love, you tap into an inner wisdom that reminds you that healing is not just about the physical body but also about nurturing your emotional, mental, and spiritual wellbeing.

By fostering a loving relationship with yourself, you create a solid foundation upon which your healing can flourish. You learn to trust your intuition, listen to your body, and honour your needs. You begin to release the limiting beliefs and stories that have held you back, replacing them with empowering truths about your resilience, strength, and potential. In doing so, your personal boundaries become much healthier.

Unlocking your healing wisdom through self-love is something that requires patience, compassion, and a willingness to show up for yourself every day. It means choosing to love yourself even when you face setbacks, challenges, and moments of doubt.

As you begin to witness the transformative power of self-love, you will start to experience a deep sense of wholeness, a connection to your authentic self, and a renewed vitality that radiates from within. You will become more resilient, more compassionate towards yourself and others, and more attuned to the wisdom that resides within you.

Let us begin this journey of self-love. To unlock the healing wisdom that lies within you. Remember, you are worthy of love, not just from others but, most importantly, from yourself. Embrace the transformative power of self-love, and watch as it paves the way for true health, wellness, and a profound connection to your inner wisdom.

Everything starts with the relationship you have with yourself.

Learning to love yourself more is the key to your healing.

Your future self will thank you for taking the responsibility to heal. You have found this book for a reason, and it is a beautiful journey of self-discovery to find out who you truly are and go through this transition. This transition is your soul coming forward and creating a new perspective of how you view yourself. Simply from the fact that you are here on the planet means you are loveable because you are created with the same energy the universe is made of, which is love.

Self-love isn't held in high regard in mainstream opinions. Self-love is even considered to be selfish which is so far from the truth as it is necessary. What starts to happen when you release trauma is that a new level of self-love starts to come into your awareness. It is deep self-love; it is a new understanding of who you are at the very core of you. You are fast-tracking yourself to be your highest version, your joyful, confident, successful, abundant self. You are starting to get to know the real you, your higher power, your true soul essence. It's not superficial, it is not relying on the labels that society has put on you. You are finding a source higher than yourself. It is a beautiful gift; you are being chosen to release those old thoughts and beliefs that society put on you. It is time to re-birth your true self. You are reclaiming your power.

# *Releasing Negative Self-Talk Patterns*

W hether you are consciously aware or not, you have that negative self-talk chatter going on in your mind. It's on autopilot, a default setting. You know the voice I mean, the one that calls you names, puts you down, makes you feel bad about yourself.

All this negative chatter is having a huge impact on your health and wellbeing. It negatively affects your mental and physical health because it is impossible to separate the mind from the body.

Whose voice is your inner critic anyway? Where did it come from? It could be from a critical parent, teacher, caregiver, or bully at school.

These negative words, thoughts, and beliefs are creating a negative charge in your body. When you start to shift and change them into more positive words, and even better, when you start believing these new beliefs, your health really starts to improve. Awareness is key. That is the first step. Now that you are aware of it, you can start to shift and change it.

Here are some suggestions for transforming your negative self-talk into empowering affirmations:

Instead of 'I'm an idiot', tell yourself:

- I am intelligent and always learning.
- Any mistakes I make are opportunities for growth.
- I am human and doing my best.
- I am imperfectly perfect just the way I am.

Replace 'I can't' with:

- I am figuring this out.
- I am capable of amazing things.
- I can do anything I put my mind to.

When your inner critic says, 'I'm not good enough', change it to:

- I am worthy and deserving of good things.
- I am loveable.
- I'm making progress every day.
- My best is always good enough.

Transform 'What if things go wrong?' to:

- I trust in my ability to handle whatever comes my way.
- I focus on positive outcomes.

- I choose faith over fear.

Some other affirmations to change negative self-talk:

- I am smart, creative and resourceful.
- I deeply love and accept myself as I am.
- Amazing opportunities are coming my way.
- I'm proud of how far I've come.
- My potential is limitless.

The words that follow 'I am' follow you and are incredibly powerful. Are you limiting yourself by your words or expanding your potential?

Remember, you are in charge of your inner dialogue. With practice, you can train your mind to support and encourage you. Be patient with the process and celebrate every time you catch and correct negative self-talk. Don't judge yourself when a negative thought pops into your head. Just be aware of it and change it, no need to blame or shame yourself. You have been doing this habit for a lifetime, so it will take time to shift, but progress is progress. Give yourself plenty of patience as you begin to become more aware of your thoughts and catch them. It takes a bit to get used to, but with perseverance, commitment, and a sincere drive to become more positive, you will be amazed at what you can achieve, and your hopes and dreams are closer than you think.

I was speaking with a friend a few days ago. She said that since she has been saying powerful affirmations such as

'I am strong', 'I am healthy', and 'I am abundant', she no longer takes medication, has lost over 2 stone in weight, improved her relationships, and generally feels so much happier. It just shows how powerful and effective this simple technique really is.

Here's your **free** Releasing Negative Self Talk Meditation for you, with love.

Meditation link

https://bit.ly/45FJ2xa

**Self-Love Mirror Work**

When you look in the mirror and see yourself, what are

your immediate thoughts?

Are your thoughts full of criticism or full of self-praise and admiration?

I bet your first thoughts are critical ones because we have all been conditioned to do that by the media and to become something that is impossible to achieve. There are many other ways we have been conditioned to go into self-hate and self-criticism such as our parents, caregivers, bullies at school, friendship groups; the list goes on.

As we discussed before, trauma disassociates you from yourself, and self-love reconnects you. It is the vital missing ingredient. Dis-ease is the dis-connection from yourself manifesting physically. This is the difference between putting the batteries in your remote the wrong way or the correct way.

Now is the time to change these patterns. It can be very simple yet very effective. Please don't be put off by the simplicity. Healing doesn't have to be complicated.

When you look in the mirror do you notice a loving, wonderful, kind loving person looking back at you? The relationship you have with yourself is the most important one. If you don't want to be with yourself, then you cannot expect real loving relationships in your life either. When you are happy and content with yourself, you will find all your relationships will improve, and the right people will want to be with you. You will find you act and react to situations differently and in a more healed way. New people will come into your life, and some may leave as your energy shifts and changes. It is an exciting journey of self-discovery.

Do this work like your life depends on it, and it can be that transformational. You have the keys to unlock your best life. Let's start unlocking the door.

The first thing I would like you to do is find some sticky notes or use some paper and poster putty that can be attached to your mirror without leaving residue.

I would like you to write positive statements on the piece of paper beginning with 'I am' because the words that follow 'I am' follow you, meaning you become what you believe to be true about yourself. They are that powerful, so it is time to make those words count.

Here's a list to start you off, and of course, you can add any more that you think of. Put about six of them on your mirror:

I am worthy, I am enough, I am perfectly imperfect just the way I am, I am clever, I am not broken but hurting and need healing, I am smart, I am successful, I am here for a reason, I matter, I am strong, I am comfortable in my body, I am happy and content being me, I am letting go of guilt, I am a good person, I am here to make my life count, I matter, I am letting in compliments now, I am allowing people I trust to become close to me, the right people like me, I belong, I am needed, I am interesting, I am loveable, I am able to take care of myself, I am finding more good people come into my life, I am calm confident and in control, I trust myself, I have amazing coping skills, I am powerful, I am bravely navigating through life's ups and downs.

Now you have a list on your mirror, stand in front of it, make eye-to-eye contact with your reflection, and repeat the phrases you have written on your mirror. Repeat them 20 times and do this every time you walk past this mirror and at least every morning and evening before you go to bed. Your mind learns by repetition, which means that you need to keep repeating these phrases often, before they become accepted as truth. Your mind has believed all the negative self-talk you have been doing over the years, so it will take a chunk of time before it accepts the new way of thinking. Remember, this does work, but you must keep practising it and make it a new good habit for life. You will see so many positive changes in your life when you make this a daily habit. Eventually, your mind will accept these beliefs more readily because you are saying them all the time.

### Inner Child Healing

It doesn't matter how old you are, there is an inner child within all of us. The inner child within you needs nurturing, feeling cared for, safe and loved. When it is safe to do so, close your eyes and imagine a mirror in front of you. In the mirror, there are all the versions of you, all the ages you have ever been reflecting back at you. Send every one of them love. Say out loud:

"I love you, I love you, I love you. You are amazing and kind, and everything was age-appropriate; you didn't know what you didn't know. I forgive you for anything you feel you need forgiving for. You are safe, you matter, and you are loved."

While you are doing this, you can also wrap your arms around yourself and give yourself a hug. That is such deep healing in itself. Repeat the words:

'You are safe, you matter, and you are loved. I love you, inner child'.

Really feel the energy and meaning behind the words as you say them. Allow all the ages you have ever been to merge and connect to you so that you feel wholeness, oneness, unity, and connection. Repeat this exercise daily, and it will give you deeper healing every time you do it.

Now, put a hand on your heart and feel the love energy within you. Allow yourself to connect to the love within you. Love is the best healing energy there is. As you connect to this love, really set the intention to feel and connect to the love within you. We all have an infinite well of love within us, it is the energy we are made from, our soul essence.

Take a deep cleansing breath in, and imagine breathing in the love. As you breathe out, imagine that you are breathing out all the energy and emotions that no longer need to be in your body. With every breath, feel the love within you increase, and the negative emotions leave your body. You can give love a colour and imagine that the colour is also getting bigger and brighter with every breath that you take. Feel that love expand beyond your physical body; feel it seep into each and every atom and cell in your body, knowing that what you are experiencing is perfect for you now. This is a beautiful exercise to reconnect to yourself and the love within you.

### Releasing Anger, Frustration, Guilt and Grief

I will now teach you how to work with your acupressure points to release frustration, anger, grief and loss.

Put your middle and index fingers of both hands to the side of your head near your eyes so that your left hand is on your left side and your right hand is on your right side. As you breathe in, focus and acknowledge any frustration. Breathe that away in two breaths and repeat four or five times until you feel a big exhale of breath.

To release grief and loss, put the index and middle finger of your right hand at the side of your left thumb. Take a deep breath in, acknowledge grief and loss as you do, and then breathe it away in a couple of exhale breaths, four or five times, until you feel a deeper exhale or a sense of release.

Pop your right index finger and middle finger onto your left index finger, at the side of it that is facing you, so that the middle finger of your right hand is at the top. Take a deep breath in acknowledging self-blame and guilt and then breathe them away in two breaths. Keep repeating four or five times until you feel calmer or feel a deeper exhalation breath.

Suppressed anger eats away at us and is the predominant emotion behind cancer, so releasing it is important. To begin, put your right hand onto your right hip and move your fingers inwards to where your liver sits, firmly press, but not too hard. Take a breath in, and as you do so, imagine or set the intention, that you are focusing on anger, and then breathe it away in two breaths. Repeat this four or five times until you feel calmer.

You can of course repeat these exercises as often as you feel you need to.

To learn more about, and release more emotions using acupressure points, take a look at Anxious to Awesome, my self-study course that is yours for life. You can also help your children release their emotions using these wonderful techniques. Knowing how to release grief was so important to me when my mum died. I remember doing this technique in a supermarket queue when a wave of grief consumed me without warning. It was very helpful. Releasing our emotions without having to be in the story of the root cause is a really gentle yet powerful and effective way to heal.

Enrol today:

http://bit.ly/3L0fNff

# The Power of Journalling Can Transform Your Life

I t can be all too easy to get caught up in the negativity and stress that surrounds us daily. However, one simple practice can help you shift your energy, take ownership of your emotions, and create the life you desire.

Gratitude journaling is the act of regularly writing down the things you are thankful for in your life. It can be as simple as jotting down a few bullet points each day or as elaborate as writing detailed entries about the people, experiences, and things that bring you joy and fulfilment. You get to choose which way is best for you.

By consistently focusing on the positive aspects of your life, you train your brain to look for the good in every situation. This shift in perspective can help you overcome challenges and maintain a more optimistic outlook. It really is life changing because where our attention goes, our energy flows.

When you take time to appreciate the things you have, you worry less about what you lack. This can lead to reduced stress levels and improved overall wellbeing.

Studies have proven that practising gratitude can significantly increase feelings of happiness and life satisfaction. By regularly acknowledging the good in your life, you cultivate a deeper sense of contentment.

Expressing gratitude to others strengthens connections and fosters more positive interactions. When you appreciate the people in your life, they are more likely to reciprocate, leading to stronger, more fulfilling relationships.

I have personally found journaling to be a game-changer. Each morning, I write down three things I wish to accomplish that day. This helps me focus my energy and prioritise my tasks. Anything that doesn't make the top three gets added to my wish list for future consideration.

In the evening, I reflect on my day and write down three things that triggered me, three things I enjoyed, and three things I can release. This practice helps me process my emotions, celebrate my successes, and release any negativity or stress accumulated throughout the day.

Laura Shofroth and I created this 10x10 Gratitude Journal in our group program now named Total Holistic Health Acceleration. There's a video embedded in the journal to really help you be in the powerful energy of gratitude, so you FEEL it, not just say the words. Our energy is the currency of the universe. Let's create gorgeous things and the life you desire together. Download it now for free.

https://bit.ly/3VFWqNg

My lovely friend Janine Kathleen Shapiro shared her method of journalling with me and has given her kind permission to share it with you too. It is taking your raw, triggered emotions into feeling calmer and more grounded and centred. Janine's method is SORE to SOAR. Here's your free link to the journal and has my video taking you

through the steps to empower yourself.

https://bit.ly/4ezoo66

## The Delight of Joy

Do you allow yourself to feel joy? Many of us who have gone through traumas believe we don't deserve joy and some of us even fear it. Remember these are just beliefs and not the real truth which means we can choose to change our beliefs at any time.

I give myself permission to feel joy now and you can too. Recently I walked from a local shop along a scenic route home. I stopped on the bridge and took in the sight and sound of the river beneath my feet.

I sat on a bench while looking at the sun. I went into an empty playground and allowed myself to swing on a swing. It was one of my happy places as a child. It felt good to feel the motion of the swing, the breeze on my face and the wind in my hair. It helped set me up for the day. Something shifted in me and I felt great all day.

What will you do today to add joy into your day? Walking in nature helps, putting your bare feet on the grass is healing and grounding at the same time.

What baby steps will you take today to give you joy? Perhaps you can receive a smile from someone you love and allow yourself to feel the joy in your heart? Perhaps you will decide to connect with your own love in your heart? Maybe you will go back to the Gratitude Journal and pick up on the energy Laura and I shared in our video that we created for you?

# *Improving Memory and Concentration*

There are several things we can do to improve our memory:

- Eat less sugar.

- Eat a healthy diet.

- Make time for meditation.

- Get enough sleep.

What is probably even more important is being consciously aware of what you tell yourself. Be mindful of your thoughts, watch what you say to yourself, and use more praise and less criticism. All of these has a massive impact on your life, your experiences and abilities, and even your memory.

What do you tell yourself?

'I have a poor memory', 'I can't remember anything', 'My memory is rubbish', 'My memory is shocking?'

Instead, start confidently declaring, 'I have a great memory!' 'It (the thing you are trying to remember) will come back to me.' 'I have an amazing memory.' 'My mind is like a search engine, it will retrieve the information in record time.'

This simple change in your self-talk can rewire your brain, boosting your ability to retain and recall information. It's a testament to the power of positive thinking and the amazing adaptability of your mind.

Imagine the possibilities that you unlock when you approach life with this optimistic, self-affirming mindset. By harnessing the power of your words, you can not only improve your memory but also enhance your overall confidence and performance.

Start reframing your thoughts and words today and notice the amazing impact it has on your life. Even better, start writing down the changes you notice. You will be amazed at the differences.

# Energy Centres Or Chakras and How to Unblock Them

F irst, let's talk about what chakras are, as it may be the first time you have come across them or know little about them. Chakras are your energy centres. You cannot see them because they are part of your energy body. They are the focus points used in a variety of ancient practises. They allow your life force energy to flow through you. They are connected to your physical, mental, emotional, and spiritual health.

Your health is affected if your energy centres become blocked or the energy isn't flowing the way it is designed to. When the chakras are flowing correctly and are in balance, they give you health, and you feel more alive. Each energy centre is associated with a colour.

There are seven main energy centres. The first is the root chakra which is located at the base of your spine and is responsible for your sense of safety and security. If this chakra is blocked, it can cause disorders of the bowel and intestines. It can also cause problems with the legs, feet, and the base of the spine. It can cause eating disorders, anxiety, depression and insecurities. All of these feed into the feeling of being powerless. The colour associated with this chakra is red. Foods that are red in colour help balance your root chakra. Some examples are carrots, tomatoes, beetroot, rhubarb and red berries.

Move your attention now up to your second chakra around 2 inches below your navel, the sacral chakra. If this energy centre is blocked, it can lead to sexual dysfunctions, problems with reproductive organs, the urinary system, constipation, muscle spasms, loss of appetite for food, sex, and life. It can make you quick to become angry. The sacral chakra is associated with the colour orange and the foods that benefit our sacral chakra are apricots, oranges, peaches and root ginger.

Moving up now to your solar plexus, your third chakra. This is located just 2 inches below your breastbone. If this energy centre is blocked, it can cause digestive disorders, depression, liver issues, diabetes, and food allergies. You may feel a lack of confidence and even a feeling that others are controlling your life. This energy centre is associated with the colour yellow. Foods such as bananas, cinnamon, chamomile, and turmeric will help to balance this chakra.

Let us move now to the fourth energy centre, the heart chakra. This energy centre is located behind the breastbone in front and on our spine between our shoulder blades on our back. As you may have guessed, it is the centre for love, compassion and spirituality. If this energy centre is blocked, it can lead to disorders of the heart and lungs, causing allergies, asthma, and circulation issues; you may feel indecisive, afraid, and unworthy of love. This is the chakra connecting body, mind and spirit. This energy centre is associated with the colour green. The foods that benefit this chakra are green vegetables such as broccoli, kale, parsley, mint, avocado, and kiwi fruits.

Now, let's focus on your fifth chakra, your throat chakra. It is in the middle of your collarbone at the base of your neck. It is the centre of communication and expression, whether in thought, speech or written words. Issues with this energy centre cause problems with our neck, teeth, throat, thyroid, parathyroid, and ears. It may make us feel we can't speak up and feel timid, quiet and weak. It is associated with the colour blue and foods that benefit this chakra are blueberries and blackberries.

Moving up to your sixth chakra, which is also known as your third eye and is located above your eyes in the centre of your forehead. If this energy centre is blocked, it can lead to headaches, ear and eye disease, nose and sinus issues, neurological disturbances and learning difficulties. This is the centre for psychic ability, higher intuition, and the energy of spirit and light. Through the power of this chakra, you can receive guidance and channel your higher self. I also think it is important to remember that your spiritual and intuitive development is developing at your unique pace, and it is not a race in spiritual development. The colour indigo is associated with this chakra. Foods that benefit this chakra are plums, figs, black grapes and red cabbage.

Let us move your attention to your seventh chakra, which is located just behind the top of the skull. It is your crown chakra. If this energy centre is blocked, it may lead to a lack of joy, feelings of frustration, migraine headaches, confusion, muddled thinking and mental disorders. This chakra is associated with the colour purple. Foods that help the crown chakra are lavender, purple onions, blackberries and blueberries.

Here is your chance to download your copy of my chakra meditation to help your chakras be balanced and flowing in their natural way.

https://bit.ly/45AVIWn

Enjoy the pleasure of just being with yourself in the moment, your chakras being more balanced, more healed and aligned. I certainly feel the shift when I listen and lots of people have told me they feel an increase in energy and feel much healthier. What will your experience be? I'd love to hear.

# *Confidence Meditation - Meeting Your Higher Self To Gain Wisdom & Answers You Seek.*

Y ou may want to record this meditation on your phone and play it back when you are relaxing in bed. Your voice is very healing to your subconscious mind.

Find a quiet, comfortable space where you can sit undisturbed for the next few minutes. Close your eyes and begin to focus on your breath. Notice the gentle rise and fall of your chest with each inhale and exhale. Allow your breath to settle into a natural, relaxed rhythm.

As you continue to breathe slowly and deeply, imagine yourself walking along a tranquil path. Feel the ground beneath your feet and the gentle breeze brushing against your skin. As you move forward, you notice a beautiful, peaceful garden ahead.

Step into this serene garden, taking in the vibrant colours of the flowers and the soothing sounds of nature around you. In the centre of the garden, you see a radiant being, it is your higher self. This is the part of you that is always connected to wisdom, love, and infinite possibility.

Approach your higher self with an open heart and mind. Notice the warmth and love emanating from their presence. As you stand before them, feel a deep sense of connection and understanding flowing between you.

Your higher self reminds you that all the answers you seek already reside within you. Trust in your intuition and inner guidance. Know that you have the strength, wisdom, and capability to navigate any challenge that comes your way.

Allow the confidence and self-assurance from your higher self to flow through you. Feel it filling every cell of your being, anchoring itself deep within you. Know that this connection to your higher self is always available to you, whenever you need it.

Take a few moments now to simply bask in the presence of your higher self and this profound connection. (Pause for 30 seconds)

As you prepare to leave the garden, thank your higher self for this experience. Know that you can return to this space anytime you need to reconnect with your inner wisdom and confidence.

Slowly retrace your steps, following the path back out of the garden. When you're ready, begin to bring your awareness back to your physical body and your breath.

Gently wiggle your fingers and toes, and when you feel grounded, open your eyes. Carry this sense of confidence and connection with your higher self throughout your day, knowing that all the answers you seek are within you.

# Ho' Oponopono Meditation

H o' oponopono is an ancient Hawaiian healing practice or technique. It is much more than just the phrases we are saying it is also the energy within the words. This is a very powerful practice, and you could record these words into your phone and use it as a daily meditation to listen to.

The basic Ho oponopono prayer is:

**I am sorry**

**Please Forgive me**

**Thank you**

**I love you**

It is traditionally recited while focusing on the person or situation you wish to forgive. It helps you clear away any emotions that are keeping you, blocking you, and holding you back from the health, money, success, or career you desire.

As we discussed throughout the book, we create our full reality. It can feel like a hard pill to swallow when we realise that we manifest and create it all. The issue(s) or situation you are experiencing has been created because there is information, beliefs, stories, and negative/training emotions that are in your system that have built up over the years or may have been inherited from ancestors and family members and are causing this disturbance in your outside world.

The good news is that as we create this ourselves, it also means we can reverse it. Release yourself of any judgment because none of it is your fault. It does mean though that you can take your power back and take responsibility to clear it, address it, and release it. Now is the time to take responsibility for clearing it up without judgment or shame.

Focus on the issue you want to support yourself in clearing. It is probably a health issue, as you are already reading this book, but it is worth remembering that it also works extremely well with your relationship with money, your success, your career, and any area of your life because you are creating everything in your outside world.

Keep in mind what issue you want to work with to clear. There is no need to know where this issue comes from or why it is there. It is enough to bring the topic to your awareness and allow yourself to feel the emotions and sensations that come up and feel them in your body.

As you think about the issue, either in your mind, or out loud, know that this is working in the background as you say these words:

I am sorry for being unaware.

I am sorry for being unaware, I didn't realise that I was creating this.

I am sorry, I have no idea where this information came from, and I don't need to know.

Please forgive me and any parts of me that have created this.

Please forgive my ancestors and family members for their part in this.

Please forgive all of us for being unaware.

Thank you, thank you, thank you, thank you, thank you, thank you.

Thank you, source/ Creator, for erasing all of this information for me.

I love you, I love you, I love you, I love you.

I am sorry for being unaware.

Forgive me, forgive my ancestors and family and all parts of me that have been creating this.

I forgive myself. There is no reason to hold on to any of this anymore.

I let it go. I drop it now. Done.

Thank you, thank you, thank you, thank you, thank you.

I love you, I love you.

Repeat four times. It is worth remembering that our higher

self doesn't hold on to things, so you can let go of them just as easily. Simply set the intention to let go.

Come back and repeat this exercise as often as you want with as many topics or issues you want to clear.

# *Decode Root Cause Method*

Over the years, my method, Decode Root Cause, has evolved and will continue to. It is a fabulous way to help you understand your personal root cause and release the emotions that are keeping you stuck in the cycle of pain and symptoms so they can be released.

I will continue to have hypnotherapy as the underlying tool because it allows the subconscious mind to come more to the forefront, and as the subconscious controls 95% of everything you do, think, feel, and believe about yourself, hypnotherapy is a fabulous gateway to work with your subconscious programming. It means that you don't need countless sessions. As hypnotherapy helped me release my daughter's autoimmune disease, it is always going to be close to my heart. We are all so quick to upgrade our laptops or mobile phones (cell phones) but often never think about updating ourselves.

This is an extremely powerful and effective method, so let's discuss what hypnotherapy is and what it isn't. Too many myths about hypnotherapy are keeping it from being utilised to its full potential.

There is a myth that a hypnotist/hypnotherapist has absolute power, command or control over the person being hypnotised. That is false. You always have the power over your thoughts and how you act and react every moment of every day.

Another myth is that hypnotised people can't resist suggestions and must follow instructions blindly. In the same way, I cannot make you give me your car keys, your money, or anything else; I cannot give you any other suggestions or beliefs you don't want. The physician lies within you. I guide you, take you to your personal roots, and expertly lead you to where you need to be to give you the best outcome possible.

Hypnosis is not something that is 'done to you' either. It is a natural state of relaxation that you go in and out of all the time. It is daydreaming or watching a film when you are absorbed in the storyline and characters. It is like driving a vehicle on a familiar road and being surprised you are further along the journey than you thought. You were thinking about other things, and your subconscious mind took over the task of driving.

Hypnosis isn't something you can get 'stuck' in either. That's like saying you can get stuck in sleep, or stuck watching a film, it simply isn't true.

A hypnotist can't make you do silly things like cluck like a chicken or perform other embarrassing tricks. Stage hypnotists look for a certain type of person who is looking and willing to perform.

Hypnosis is…

*Daydreaming*

*Driving on a familiar road* where your subconscious mind takes over and you consciously think about something else, like what you are having for dinner or a recent conversation.

*Watching a movie or TV* when you respond to how the characters feel and not wondering how many takes it took or where the director stood.

*It is a transitional state between being awake and asleep.* You naturally enter this state every time you go to bed.

*It is a natural state of relaxation.* You're fully conscious and aware of your surroundings. You are simply relaxed, that means that you are more in your subconscious mind, which is the emotional part of your mind and where memories are stored. This is the perfect state to explore your personal root cause of the issue you want to work with so it can be healed and released, whether it is emotional or physical. Your subconscious mind knows how, when, where and why it began. Your subconscious controls at least 95% of everything you think, feel and believe about yourself.

The very nature of working with your subconscious means

it is far more effective than traditional talk therapy and is likely to achieve long-lasting results more quickly. The conscious mind will not know the answers, but the subconscious mind will. That is why talking therapies aren't as effective, or take lots of sessions. Hypnotherapy is more relaxing.

I help relax you simply by talking to you and allowing you to relax your body and mind by listening to my voice.

Every state of hypnosis is self-hypnosis. It cannot be done 'to you'. It is simply a natural state of relaxation that you choose to be in.

If 'blind obedience' was a true phenomenon there would be many more millionaire hypnotherapists because they'd be instructing their clients to give them all their money. If I asked you for your car keys in any conversation, you would simply reject the idea and say no.

Instead of a sleepy state, hypnosis is a heightened state of awareness. We naturally enter and exit this state all the time.

When you are relaxed, your subconscious mind is more prominent, with your conscious mind drifting off. Relaxation calms that critical filter factor, which means that you are more open to more powerful, positive suggestions. You can upgrade old thought patterns that hurt you and replace them with more positive, helpful thoughts and beliefs.

We discover your personal reason, plan, aim, and goal for why the issue you want to resolve exists and work to release any resistance to change and the motivational part that brought you in front of me to help you get the best outcome possible, in as few sessions as possible.

How effective is hypnotherapy?

Alfred A Barrios, Ph. D, presented a review in the journal *Psychotherapy Theory, Research and Practice* and in *American Health* magazine.

There, he provided the following success rates: psychoanalysis, an average of 600 sessions to give 38% success rate; behaviour therapy, an average of 22 sessions to give 72% success rate; and hypnotherapy, an average of 6 sessions to give 93% success rate.

The results speak for themselves.

# *Conclusion*

T hank you for taking this healing path with me. Some of the things we discussed were what trauma is and how it is not so much what happened to us but how these events affect our view of ourselves, how trauma fragments us from our true soulful selves and impacts us in every moment, although we are often unconscious of it.

I created a list of ailments and symptoms, and although not an exhaustive list, I hope you can begin to understand how our body speaks the truth, and its language is pain and symptoms. I hope you can also start to see the meaning behind each body part where the symptoms occur.

I shared my story so you can see what's possible for you when we heal at the root and how, because I may have gone through something similar, I can hold that safe space for you to heal and release too.

I hope you found the 'Unlock the Wisdom to Heal' section very insightful and are willing to implement these tips and techniques into your daily practice. They may look like simple practices, but don't let that fool you into thinking they aren't powerful because they truly are. You can think of it as life before you read this book and life after; it really can be that life-changing.

If you are looking for deeper healing to unlock your unique personal root cause without countless sessions take a look at my website for more information or send me an email. I would love to welcome you to my free Facebook group 'Decoding The Body's Messages To Transform and Thrive'

I look forward to hearing from you.

Much love

*Rachel*

For free resources, meditations to release anxiety, balancing your energy centres, listen to my podcast where clients share their experience of working with me, download my testimonial ebook Transform & Thrive in the 'free gift' section, learn more about my group programs, working with me 1:1, group programs and more, please visit my website:

www.wellnesswithrachel.co.uk

All details are on my website or email me at:

rachel@wellnesswithrachel.co.uk

Join my Facebook group:

https://www.facebook.com/groups/
decoding.the.bodys.messages.transform.and.thrive

# *Acknowledgement*

There have been so many people supporting me with this book you know who you are.

Thank you to all of the cheerleaders along the way, You have no idea how important your words of encouragement have been.

Thank you to you, the reader, as without you the book would have had no purpose.

Special thanks to Authors & Co for your help and guidance.

I love and appreciate you all.

# About The Author

## Rachel Claire Farnsworth

Rachel is a multi-award-winning Trauma Releasing Specialist, Transformational Coach and Wellness Therapist who has transformed the lives of thousands of people around the world.

In her groundbreaking debut book, Rachel takes you on an empowering journey towards your true self-love, the ultimate antidote to trauma.

Rachel reveals how our past experiences shape false beliefs that burden us with feelings of abandonment, rejection, and more. Learn to understand pain and symptoms as essential messages your body is sending you, each telling a deeper story.

By addressing these messages, Rachel helps you reconnect with your true self, allowing for profound healing and vitality. She unpacks the idea that trauma causes disassociation while true self-love bridges the gap, bringing you back to a state of wholeness and wellness.

Rachel's daughter was diagnosed with an autoimmune disease and was the catalyst for Rachel's dedication to wellness. Her daughter's recovery stands as a testament to the powerful healing techniques shared within these pages.

www.ingramcontent.com/pod-product-compliance
Lightning Source LLC
Chambersburg PA
CBHW071858200326
41519CB00016B/4439